SLEEP GUIDE

THE MENTAL AND ANCESTRAL SLEEP GAME

MASTERED

By: Kurt Yazici

Printed in the United States of America

First Printing, 2020

Cover Art by Cedric Mendoza
Interior Book Design by Ingrid Seballos

TABLE OF CONTENTS

1. FOREWORD

Scientists and researchers today are just now beginning to understand the complexity of sleep. As such an important aspect of human health and physical optimization, it has been a truly rewarding topic to research and master for my body and mind.

I've tracked 100's of nights and tested countless variables in a quest to determine the biggest variables impacting sleep quality. Even today, I'm still learning methods and approaches to helping people deal with sleep challenges to improve their routine and sleep quality.

Optimal sleep is arguably **THE SINGLE BIGGEST LEVER** of peak human performance. So why would one ever not take the time to master this area we spend 1/3 of our lives in?

In these pages, I've compiled some of the best, most cutting edge, leading info on what is known about sleep science and energy optimization. Herein lie some of the best practices I've synthesized all in one place on how one can better understand, improve, and completely optimize sleep.

I've taken a complex and often misunderstood topic and made it simple for even the most uninformed sleeper to better understand.

I encourage you to read this and take control of your sleep. You will undoubtedly rest easier and feel more energized after mastering the sections laid out in this book.

Kurt Yazici

2. INTRODUCTION

Welcome! This is a culmination of everything I've learned about sleep and how I've optimized it to support a busy, athletic, high-functioning CEO lifestyle.

I will share my personal story battling insomnia and coming out of it. Though our journeys to this point may differ, the destination of our sleep we have is the same. I believe we all want optimized, efficient, deeply restorative sleep, setting us up to be our very best mentally and physically, every single day.

Of all the books and articles on sleep I came across almost none mentioned the mental aspect. What are you supposed to think about when you're lying awake? How do you deal with the anxious sensations building when you can't fall asleep? What about the years of poor sleep, that now support a limiting belief that you can no longer sleep deeply and restoratively?

I believe this critical aspect is overlooked and poorly addressed in the current literature. Though some of the authors may have direct experience, many of the writers are researchers, not guides. Many have never journeyed through endless months of insomnia, lying awake for hours, angry, frustrated, afraid, and emotionally stuck desiring optimal sleep.

So many people have lost their belief that they can sleep deeply and soundly throughout the night. They've submitted to a concept that poor sleep is a "life-sentence" from which they will never escape.

Sleeping 7.5-9 hours throughout the night, deeply, peacefully and restfully is completely outside their reality. According to the CDC, nearly 1/3 of Americans are not getting adequate sleep. [...]

As with any gradual erosion, the damage of poor, limited sleep, can often take years to surface. Maybe at first, one just starts waking up earlier without being able to fall back asleep. Then after weeks of this, it's no longer a random event but the new status quo. Your mind expects it, your conscious self anticipates it. Before you know it, you've imprinted upon your deeper mind a new belief that you cannot fall back asleep.

In this book, we will go into this "mind game" of sleep. We will explore it deeply together.

For many, impressing direct subconscious affirmations (which at first may feel and seem far-fetched) can make a drastic improvement. But I assure you, your belief system is extremely powerful at taking control.

One thing I've realized is that we humans are incredibly powerful intellectuals. Evolution has gifted us with the largest brains to body mass, and these organs contain incredible powers beyond our waking awareness. When you sleep, you tap into other aspects of your mind.Interesting to note, some of the greatest thinkers: Thomas Edison, Albert Einstein, Sir Issac Newton and Aristotle, among several others, were all notorious nappers. They realized the power of accessing their entire minds. They would frequently tap into the creative functions of their minds by drifting in and out of states of wakefulness.

Interestingly *Edison believed that through the invention of artificial light, he could eliminate the need for human sleep. Back in the late 1800s, and early 1900s, we knew so much less than we do now! My goal is for us to have this intellectual scope ALONG WITH physical power.*

The Map of this Book

Jim Kwik, a famous speed reader, memory trainer and learning coach, taught me something critically important. We are taking a journey every time we begin a book. Having a map before embarking on a new journey will always improve your travel. It's the first step to a well-planned trip. Let's briefly cover where we'll be going in this book.

We'll start with my story of how I became so interested in sleep (Chapter 3). As a budding entrepreneur, I gave myself anxiety and insomnia as my companies and staff grew. I didn't know much about these disorders and struggled at first to manage it all. This eventually forced me on the journey of facing those challenges and better educating myself in these areas of health.

I first dug deep into anxiety, which then led me to trauma. After getting severe insomnia, I really started learning about sleep. Books such as The Sleep Revolution, Why We Sleep, The Power of When, Sleep by Littlehale, and Alex Fergus's Ultimate Guide, all primed my sleep knowledge. Blogs from Oura Ring and Whoop Band biotracker devices have further enhanced my personal experience and sleep understanding.

From these resources, I'll provide a brief anatomy of sleep (Chapter 4), and then we'll transition into sleep importance (Chapter 5). We'll discuss sleep benefits and what we currently know.

We'll dive into one of my favorite topics, the conscious mental approach to sleeping better (Chapter 6). We'll spend detailed time outlining methods that I've found over the years to be some of the most crucial elements to optimizing sleep.

We'll journey into priming our bodies (Chapter 7), looking at and better understanding all the physical things we can do to enhance our body's ability to optimally sleep.

We won't stop there though, we have a lot of ground to cover, and we'll continue our journey into sleep environment fundamentals (Chapter 8), diving into WHEN we should sleep (Chapter 9). Many of you may be messing up your flow by staying up too late OR even going to bed TOO early.

We'll end our journey discussing the best bedtime rituals for sleep preparation (Chapter 10) and finally covering the best accessories, supplements, and aides to get you resting incredibly (Chapter 11).

So if you're ready, let's begin!

3. BACKSTORY

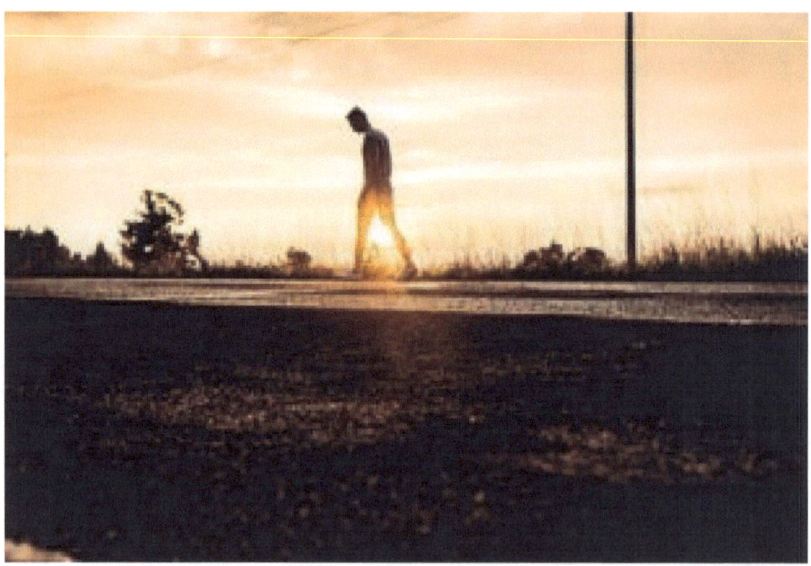

Image source: https://stuartluce.com/2018/04/29/serving-relationships-that-bless/

Most of my life, I'd never had an issue falling or staying asleep at night. It wasn't until I became a CEO leading large teams that I started experiencing challenges sleeping. Up until that point, I could always easily fall asleep, sleeping deeply and soundly throughout the night.

But once I left my corporate career in my early 30s, stress immediately amplified with added responsibilities. The gap between what I could mentally and emotionally handle, and my abilities to handle it, grew. My company quickly outgrew my skills. Mentally I suffered, due to poorly mishandling all that was happening. Ruminating, focusing on the negative, forcing, instead of unplugging, lead to serious sleep challenges.
I'd never valued sleep nor prioritized it. It was an obstacle to be hurdled when possible. I'd developed a habit of using stimulants to boost myself back to baseline. I'd also developed an anxiety disorder that directed my focus on the negatives of work, and fed a challenging cycle. As the cycle escalated, it became difficult to even get through a day.

The mounting negative emotions were consistently reaggravated by failed projects and dire financials in my businesses. At the time, I was in a business partnership and relationship, where communication had eroded irreparably. I found myself an anxious wreck that knew very little about how to cope with, and better manage the situation.

The Death of My Sleep

About 2 years into the entrepreneurial world, I found myself consistently struggling to fall asleep. Nightly, I'd lay down and my heart would start racing, anxious emotions would fill my body and feed a racing mind. Eventually, the cycle built to a point where I was no longer worrying about the challenges of the day, but was entirely focused on whether or not I was actually going to fall asleep, and sleep well.

Anxious nights of insomnia were dreadful. Dark, scary, and completely isolating for long agonizing hours. I'd lay wide awake in bed with my eyes closed, often angry and frustrated, dreading the time I'd wake up feeling exhausted, not rejuvenated and rested.

Like showing up for an exam having not properly studied, the activity of sleeping felt hopeless.

Those nerves forged a cycle that had me staying up all night laying in bed. I'd get angry and frustrated at myself and my mind, trying to channel and change my thinking, control my thoughts or think about "relaxing" and "calming" things. It became common to have days of feeling exhausted, tired and defeated because I had not slept the night before.

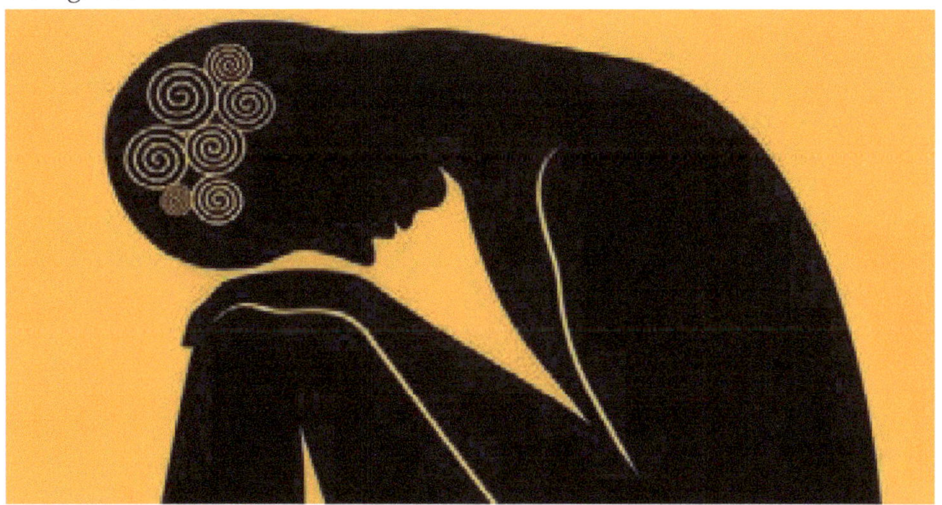

Bad Coping

If you've ever studied anxiety, one of the ways it manifests is through habits of avoidance. Individuals struggling with anxiety avoid anything and everything that triggers it. The silver lining with insomnia is you can't avoid sleeping; you must eventually succumb to it.

I developed anxiety about the idea of sleeping. Everything I did leading up to sleep would make me more anxious. I'd be extremely careful not to "upset" or deviate from my routine. A late night dinner, and I'd psych myself into an anxious fit and almost always struggle to fall asleep. Eat something, do something outside my routine, and I came to expect a harsh case of insomnia. I felt trapped and stuck. I was scared to do anything in the evenings that would trigger insomnia.

It was brutal, and it felt unbeatable. Sleepless nights can be very quiet, lonely, long and agonizing. If you've ever been there, I know exactly what it's like. But I have also learned to and know what it's like to sleep deeply, recover totally, and to be totally confident that I can fall asleep quickly and easily every night without challenge. I can go to bed with thoughts of joy and peace. I can sleep deeply and soundly throughout the whole night. Whether I'm traveling, out late, in bed early, my conscious confidence in my ability to sleep is incredible.

At this point you may be saying "yeah okay, but you don't understand me.. I've been dealing with x.. I've had this all my life.." And I hear you, but follow along, I realize it can feel impossible. But it's not, you can conquer this.

I'm in several sleep mastermind groups and I frequently average much higher DEEP and REM sleep numbers compared with others. I share this to **impress upon you** that you can go from a struggling insomniac, to someone who has control over your ability to fall asleep and sleep exceptionally. If you read this book and implement these concepts, you will sleep incredibly well and take back your natural ability to recover and feel fully rested. Mastering this will have a profound impact on your quality of your days.

The Recovery

After a year of battling insomnia, I began heavily researching and looking for answers to what was happening. I read a number of books and took several seminars on the topic. In my learning, I developed several habits, and I am confident this book will give you all you need to sleep soundly and awaken feeling refreshed. I see beautiful dreams and great ZZZs in your near future!

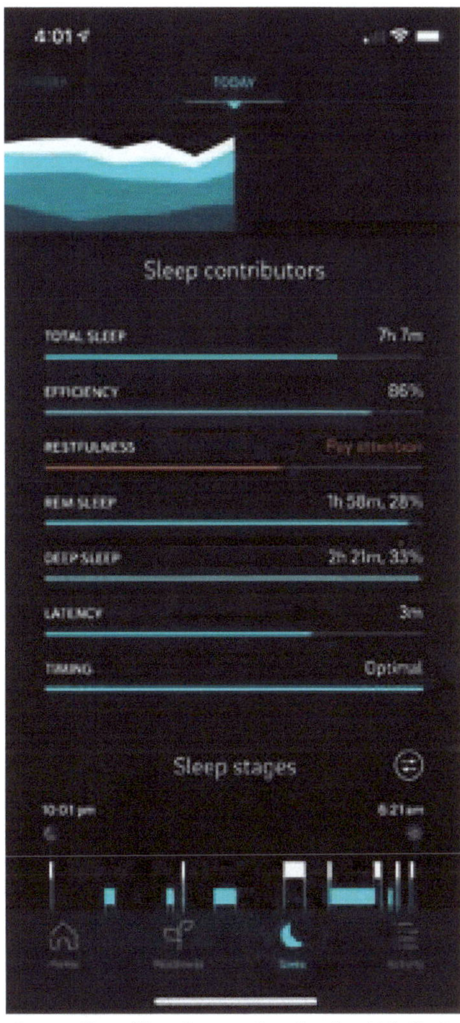

Image: Oura Ring sleep tracker showing high % & levels of REM and Deep sleep.

I want you to not only sleep better, but have a war chest of tools that will absolutely destroy those anti-sleep demons. Reading this book and implementing the recommended actions is going to leave you completely confident in your ability to sleep deeply and refreshingly each and every night, even in the most challenging and stressful life situations.

Whether you've experienced chronic exhaustion and insomnia for years, or just recently started having restless nights, the sections below will lead you to the promised land of beautiful, peaceful, satisfying, deep rest and recovery.

In the next section, we're going to view the high level of what sleep is, why it's essential and then we'll get into the keys to improving it.

4. ANATOMY OF SLEEP

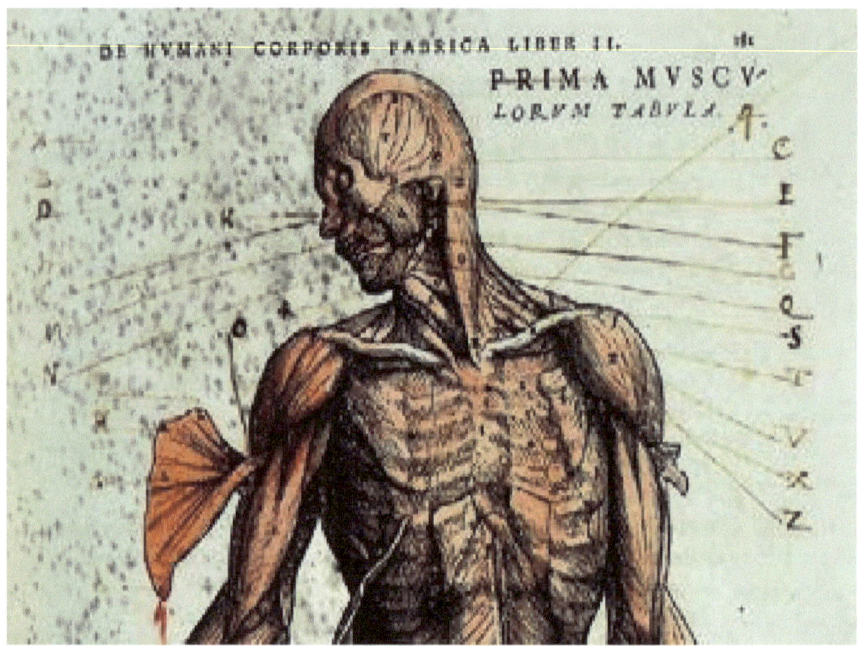

Image: https://www.nature.com/articles/d41586-018-05941-0

To sleep better, we'll take a quick, high level tour of the different stages of sleep. The American Association for Sleep Medicine (AASM) categorizes sleep into five distinct stages. [1] For our purposes, we're going to focus on the three below and **exclude wakefulness and relaxed wakefulness** as they are less of what we think of when considering our "sleep."

A. Light Sleep
B. Deep Sleep: Slow Wave
C. REM Sleep: Dreaming

A. Light Sleep

For most healthy adults, this is where you spend the majority of nightly sleep time. It is a stage of light, regenerating sleep. You experience rest and recuperation as muscles relax. That said, most sleep experts agree Deep and REM are much more valuable stages to optimize for.

Light sleep happens throughout the night and, at no particular time more than another.

B. Deep Sleep

Deep sleep is thought of as the fountain of youth.

This is a slow-wave sleep where the body and brain do a lot of physical repair. Your brain's glymphatic system removes waste and neurotoxins. Your muscles and body recover, releasing human growth hormone (HGH) to repair and build back up the damage from daily exercise and activity. During this stage, your eyes do not move. Heart rate and blood pressure will decrease and slow down. It is difficult to wake up from this stage as you're about as offline as you can be.

Deep sleep tends to occur more towards the beginning of the night. If you stay up later than usual, you'll typically see a dramatic drop in overall deep sleep, while earlier bedtimes usually support longer intervals.

Side Note - *As you'll learn later, sleep timing is a powerful lever to improve or wreck sleep quality.*

C. REM Sleep

Rapid Eye Movement (REM) is a powerful stage where our brains file and process the day's learnings and memories. We hear about this sleep because it most directly correlates with dreaming and often occurs near the end of the night, right before we're waking. Your body is paralyzed during this stage, and interestingly, is a unique sleep stage only mammals experience from the animal kingdom. REM sleep is significantly longer in humans than in other animals, and many believe it's due to our superior cognitive abilities.

It's generally thought that we want to optimize sleep as much as possible for Deep and REM sleep. The more of those two stages we get, the more physically and mentally rested we will feel. Ironically our Deep sleep occurs mostly when we get to bed early and our REM sleep occurs largely when we don't wake too soon. As we'll learn, cutting either of these may negatively impact getting sufficient amounts and properly resting.

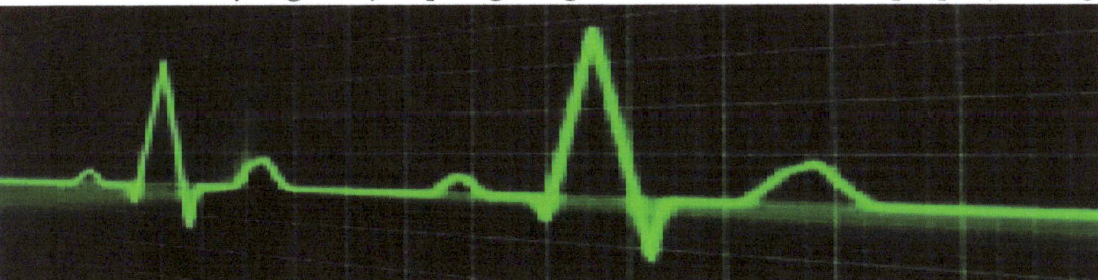

Image: https://www.networkworld.com/article/3194784/network-check-ups-critically-important-to-a-business-health.html

5. IMPORTANCE OF SLEEP

Don't worry if this section is frustrating, I felt much the same way. I realize for many of you, the value of sleep is already extremely clear and you realize the benefits and experience you get from optimal sleep. But let's clarify and **strengthen our WHY** so we all have the proper and sufficient motivation to travel this road to overcoming our less than optimal sleep.

Sleep is without question a key to living greatly. It is the ultimate cognitive enhancing nootropic. It is the ultimate physical performance enhancer. It is the best way to treat and prevent disease and health deterioration.

If you get it right, in the right amount and quality, **you WILL perform significantly better.** You will transform your entire life in all areas. The effects are deep and long-term for your health and disease prevention.

Unfortunately, perception of sleep quality is highly subjective.

Sleep-deprived individuals have extremely poor conscious interpretations of how well they are performing. Similar to a drunk person whose judgment is horribly impaired and yet thinks they can operate a vehicle well, sleep-deprived humans are often unaware of what optimal sleep truly is.

The objective reality is much different than the subjective. Sleep deprivation is one of the largest causes of car accidents.[2]

Imagine slowly becoming more unknowing, becoming more intoxicated as you attempt to perform in your job, at the gym and in your relationships. The quality of your life and intelligence would undoubtedly decline.

How well you perform and the quality of your life are directly supported by your sleep. *The irony of bad sleep and insomnia is our inability to objectively realize how bad our performance is.*

Major benefits of optimal sleep include:

1. Sharper Cognition [3] [4] [5] [6] [7] [8]
2. Improved Mood [9] [10] [11]
3. Healthier Heart [12]
4. Athletic Performance [13] [14]
5. Cancer Prevention [15]
6. Stress Reduction [16]
7. Inflammation Reduction [17] [18]
8. Improved Alertness [19]
9. Improved Memory [3] [4] [5] [6] [8]
10. Weight Loss [20] [21]
11. Physical Recovery [22]

This list goes on MUCH further; we could fill chapters with clear references. Needless to say, as we optimize through the tips below, we're going to see dramatic and significant impacts on our lives.

Even if you don't want to change your social schedule, diet, or implement any number of the recommendations below, simply **increasing sleep quality is powerful.** With even a few of these improvements, ratcheting up sleep quality by small increments can compound the effect sleep will have on the rest of your life.

> "*EVEN if you do nothing to increase and/ or change the times you sleep, the benefits you'll see with just a few tweaks below are going to improve your sleep QUALITY and efficiency dramatically, hence the overall experience of life and health.*"

This short section was dense. There were a lot of references and studies. You don't need to know or remember them. All I ask is that you keep close, the concept that sleep is about as important a lever in your overall well-being, performance, and life experience as anything.

Now that we've gone through the basics, it's time to get to work on improving sleep! Let's carry on to the one of the most powerful, and frankly poorly covered topics for sleep.

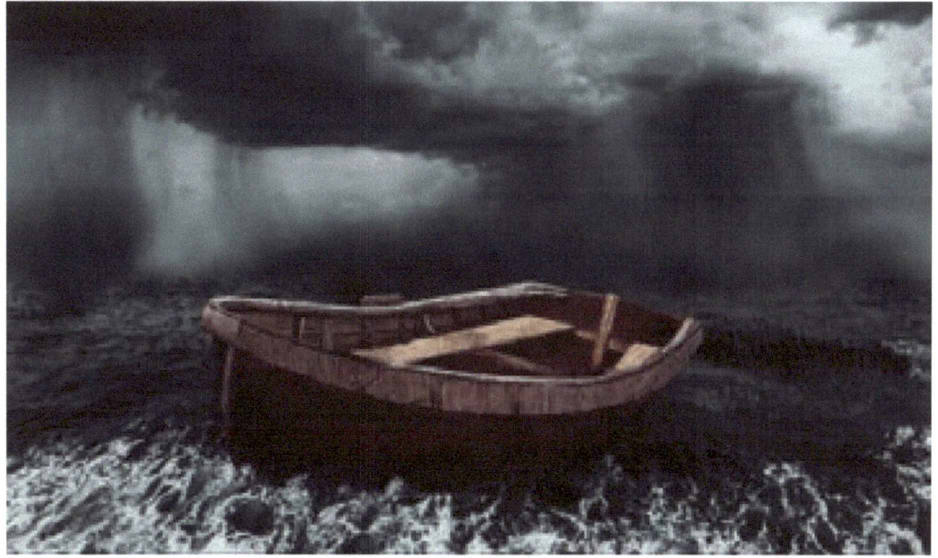

6. CONDITIONING THE MIND FOR OPTIMAL SLEEP

Almost all books on sleep address the **physical outer hygiene** aspects of sleep (we will cover that in detail below), without truly diving into practical tips on "how to" handle the mind and deal with thinking around insomnia. I've read a number of books and articles, and rarely have I found much.

I believe this section will be incredibly powerful for many of you, as it certainly was for me. The mindset of optimal sleeping was something that took me a great deal of time to refine and hone. So much of sleeping soundly and deeply is a mental game.

"Whether you think you can or you can't, you're right." Henry Ford

Brain activity during sleep does not shut off. You instead drift out of conscious alertness into different phases. You're not turning off your mind during sleep, but instead shifting into other parts of it. Because of this, I believe it's crucial to focus on unconscious programming impressions to aid and fuel deep-rooted beliefs supporting optimal sleep.

Without active development of empowering unconscious beliefs, consistent negative thought patterns can have a profound effect on your sleep quality. The cycle reinforces itself as you keep going through consistently rough nights of poor sleep. Consciously you wake feeling tired, stressed, moody, and you begin to expect it. It is a brutal self-fulfilling prophecy of poor sleep consistently reinforced.

A. Sleep Affirmations

This may sound a bit woo woo, but bare with me. One of the things we need to keep in mind is that beliefs are ingrained ways we view our world in our subconscious minds. You have to respect that a lot of what you experience and anticipate day to day is being driven by a **deeper part of you, COMPLETELY outside your conscious awareness**. Retaking control over that requires conditioning that part of your mind with new beliefs.

Feeling doubtful? Are we going against some of your beliefs right now? Realize that your body will signal emotions of doubt when you lack certainty, when you lack alignment in what you're consciously processing and what you unconsciously believe.

Rewriting Bad Programming

Written affirmations are a powerful way to reprogram your subconscious. When you write down well-formulated present-tense, directed statements, repeatedly, you impress a new focus. Day by day, night by night, you condition your deeper mind to focus on what you want to believe.

For many of us, this means rewriting beliefs and thoughts outside our conscious awareness that are sabotaging our efforts for restful, joyful regenerative sleep.

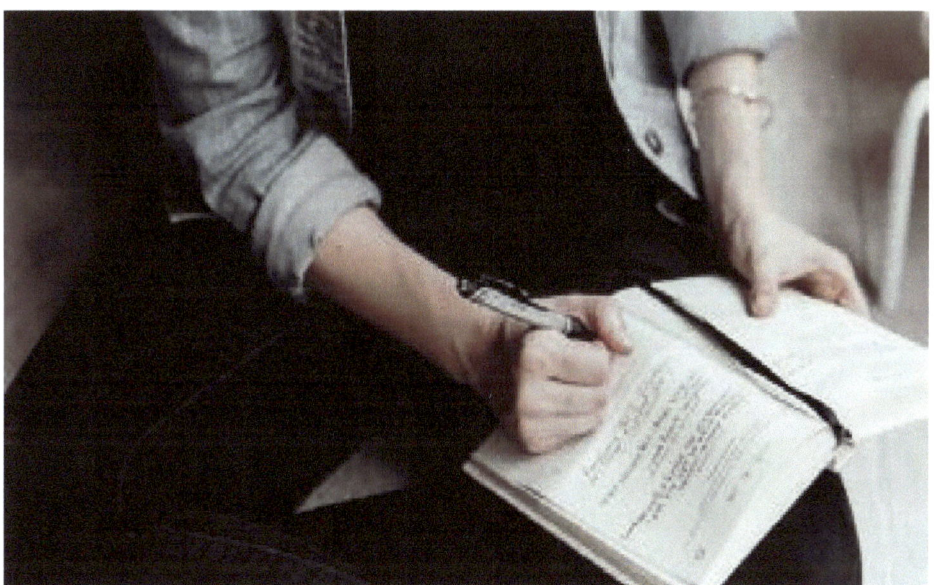

Directing Towards

The mind is firing off over 30,000 thoughts a day. Many of them are outside our awareness, but we can rewrite the record and get new programming in. We can begin to reinforce the new beliefs that support our new reality that sleeping deeply is not just a fantasy but something we experience each night; all throughout our nights, easily, peacefully and restfully.

To do this, you simply need to state the affirmation in the positive and remember to use present vs. future tense. Give the mind a point of focus, do not tell the mind where you don't want to go. Instead, tell it where you are.

Do not tell the mind where you don't want to go. Instead, tell it where you are.

Good vs. Bad Affirmations

"I will not have a bad night of sleep" This example uses negation and future tense, "not" and is focusing on what **you don't want**, rather than what you do want and are experiencing now. The mind is designed to focus in a direction, so always state affirmations in the direction you want.

"*I sleep deeply and soundly*" is an example where you are stating where you want to go and what you want to focus on right now.

Future vs. Present Tense

The other big mistake people often make with affirmations that I touched on above is they state them in the future. In theory, they sound great, "*I will have a wonderful night sleep..*" The problem is if you're constantly programming the mind to say "I will" it will consistently be repeating a message that it will come in the future instead of happening right now. You program the unconscious of expecting it in the future, but not actually experiencing it now.

> Good vs. bad examples of tense use:
> Bad: "I will sleep deeply and soundly.."
> Good: "I sleep deeply and soundly.."

The words 'I' vs. "you" can be used interchangeably as long as they have meaning to you, that you are talking about yourself. Most affirmations are stated as 'I' but they can also be stated with "you." The main area where I've seen "you" used is in times of "mirror work."

Mirror Work

Louise Hay was an incredible thinker in the field of self-healing, and she wrote some powerful writings about Mirror Work. [23] She's the founder of Hay House [24] which has published an enormous number of books in the field of self-help, many around conditioning your mind, and healing your body.

Mirror work is essentially looking yourself in the eyes through a mirror and stating positive, reinforcing, "build-you-up" incantations and affirmations.

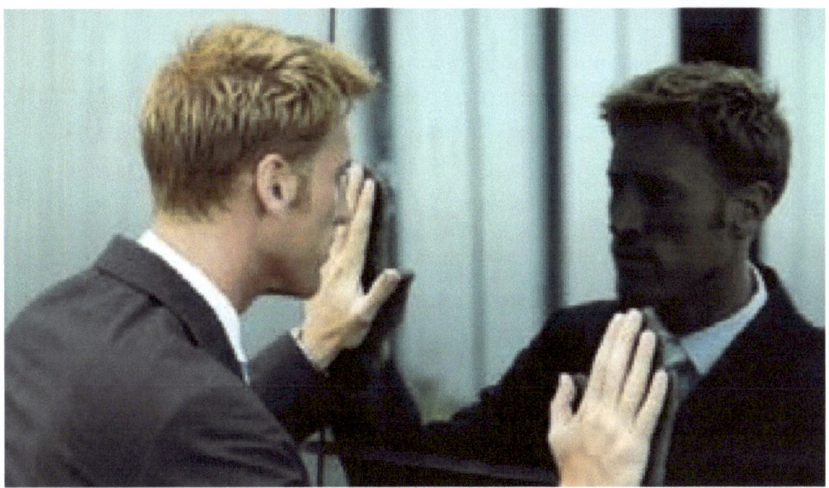

Image: Self affirmations - Mirror work

With mirror work, you develop your affirmations and then simply practice repeating them, typically 3-7 affirmations, 5-10 times each in the mirror while looking into your eyes.

Written Work

With written work, you keep a hand-written or digital journey and repeatedly write down or type your affirmations. Writing 3-5 statements 3-5 times in repeated fashion seems to be the optimal amount for most.

Both methods are powerful, and with a daily morning and evening practice of just a few minutes, you can create a dramatic change in a couple of weeks.

Affirmations

So what are the affirmations that work best? Well, I think it will differ depending on the individual, but here are a few of my favorite sleep ones (you can steal). I used to write these down nightly for months while I was working on reprogramming limiting beliefs:

1. I sleep deeply and soundly all throughout the night, awakening bright and re-freshed
2. I fall asleep quickly, easily, peacefully and happily.
3. Sleeping deeply and restfully comes easily and naturally to me.
4. Whenever I lay down, calmness washes over me.
5. Falling asleep comes naturally and easily to me.

*You can add more variations of these with words by changing 'I' -> "You" and inserting "always" after those pronouns. Go with what feels best for you at the time, and if you feel you need to, change them up after 7-10 days of practice.

> *"I sleep deeply and soundly all throughout the night, awakening bright and refreshed.*
> *I fall asleep quickly, easily, peacefully and happily.*
> *Sleeping deeply and restfully comes easily and naturally to me.*
> *Whenever I lay down, calmness washes over me.*
> *Falling asleep comes naturally and easily to me."*

B. Directing Conscious Physical Focus

Another technique I found incredibly powerful, especially when getting anxious while lying down and not falling asleep right away is **focusing**.

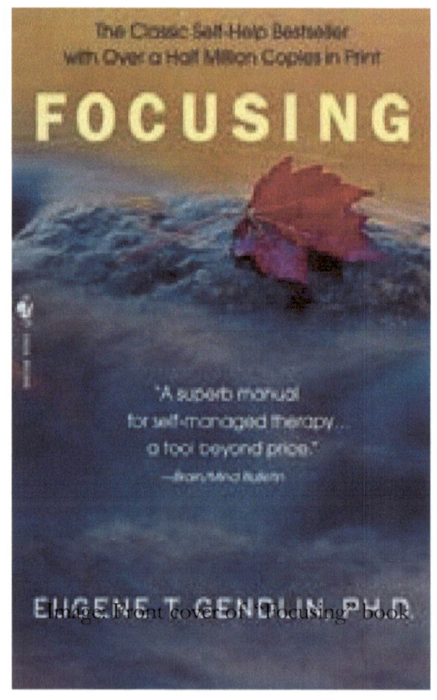

Image: Front cover of "Focusing" book

My body physically creates anxiety by building tension near my heart and neck area. Kind of scary areas, we all manifest stress and resistance in different ways. I'd prefer it elsewhere, but that's the way it manifests for me physically. Eventually, if I continue to focus on those sensations, they grow in intensity and my cognitive mind starts losing control. My logic, rational self shuts down, and the sensations start taking over activating more of my primal nerves and instincts.

In his book Focusing, Eugene Gendlin explains how emotions are created and held in the body. He explains how focusing on sensations without defining them into an emotion creates separation.

Through becoming more objective and aware, we can shift those feelings. As an example, the sensations between anxiety and excitement are often quite similar. The intensity and location of the sensations, as well as what we mentally label them can have a large impact on how we interpret them.

Emotions are actually familiar combinations of physical sensations generated by the body in specific locations. Nervousness and excitement at the sensation level are often extremely similar, but will have slight differences in intensity and location within the body.

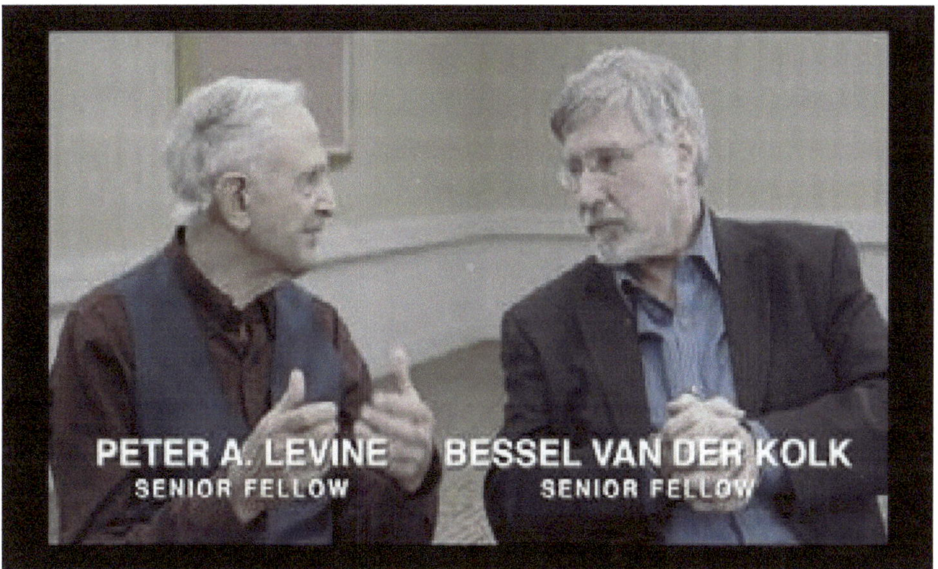

Image: Peter Levine and Bessel Van Der Kolk

From studying Focusing and the trauma works of Peter Levine [..] and Bessel Van Der Kolk [..], I've learned that when I'm laying down and I start to focus on feelings of sensations of anxiety without awareness and objectivity, they will intensify. As the well-known saying goes.

"Energy flows where focus goes" Tony Robbins.

If I'm dealing with sensations that lead to anxious emotions, then my mind starts to develop anxious thoughts. This cycle if unchecked or misunderstood, can often build and magnify the emotion. If not interrupted, the mind can trigger the body to produce adrenaline and cortisol, which no longer supports drifting off into a peaceful sleep.

If I can separate or shift the focus away from those feelings, I can short-circuit the loop of anxiety or any other negative emotion. The mantra "where focus goes, energy flows" has wisdom we can learn to harness.

Next time something like this happens - a powerful thing you can do is direct your conscious focus to another part of your body where you feel calm and relaxed.

For most of us, the tips of our toes and bottoms of our feet or hands are not areas where negative emotions manifest. So for me, that's exactly where I go if I find my mind racing and I have enough awareness to redirect my focus. The chest and heart may pound. The heart and stomach may feel out of sorts, but if you can direct your attention to other parts of your body, energy and sensations in the chest, heart and stomach areas will subside and lose their momentum.

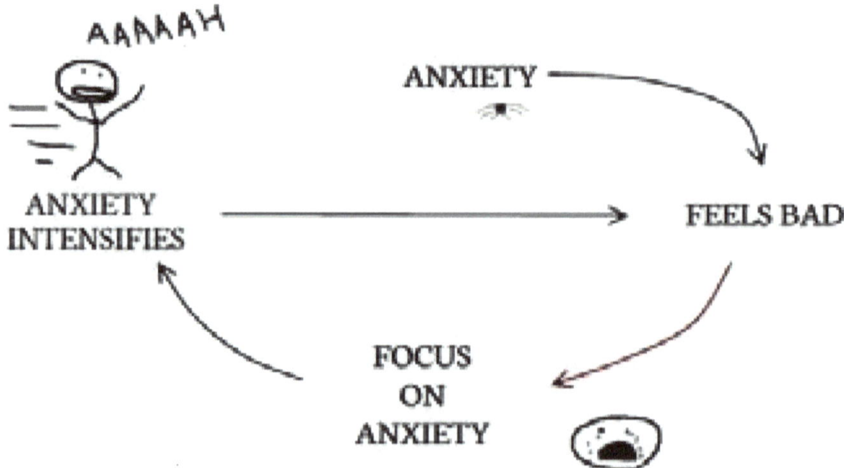

Image Source: https://www.walkingoncustard.com/laughing-at-anxiety/

Personally focusing on my feet, and staying there despite experience sometimes even growing sensations elsewhere that link with the feelings of anxiety will negatively impact me. This is also a powerful way.

C. What to Think About While Falling Asleep

Repeated practice of affirmations will create unconscious momentum and will create an undercurrent of thoughts supporting your conscious goals. Going to sleep when you lay down will become faster and more peaceful, if you practice them for weeks consistently. But what do you think about at that exact moment when you're falling asleep?

As you'll learn through the following sections, when you set your physical self up properly, and you now have these above tools for programming your unconscious and catching anxiety loops, falling asleep will become much easier no matter what you do.

But, the one RULE about thinking that I have learned, is that I rarely ever think about sleep, or anything related to insomnia while falling asleep. What I've found most effective is to let your thoughts drift, to space out and let your mind go where it wants without trying to control or be aware of your thinking (while avoiding any insomnia, worry, fear type thinking). While spacing out try and see visually in your mind the details of the thoughts and memories.

Minding Yourself to Sleep

I've learned through practice that this is one of the most effective ways to confidently drift to sleep quickly. Letting go of your mind, your awareness of your mind's thinking, and go deep into whatever it is bringing visually. This could be an experience, memory, skill. Usually it is something you directly did that you're rewatching in your mind from the day prior. If you master this what you'll find is your body naturally relaxes deeply right before you slip into slumber and the time it takes you to get there can be very short. (Often a few mins at most) Careful though, noticing when you fall asleep will often pull into consciousness which will disrupt your drift into sleep.

If you're struggling with this then focus on feelings of coziness, safety and comfort. When I feel those primal feelings of safety, and pepper in and direct myself to thoughts of neutral things, thoughts of gratitude or thoughts of love - it's in those moments I also cross over to the stages of sleep.

If I ruminate and focus on thoughts of concerns, thoughts of insomnia in the past, thoughts of overcoming insomnia in the future, I can get caught in a loop that leads to thoughts that can mess with my ability to fall asleep in the moment.

Thinking when falling asleep is a strange thing. I've journalled for months and tried to catch the exact thoughts when I've fallen asleep, but I am never able to consciously recall them. My mind will often drift into neutral thoughts, recent interactions, emotional points from the day, problems (not fearful thoughts) I'm wrestling with to find solutions.

It's okay to allow yourself to think about those things, as I mentioned above the thought to avoid is thinking about sleep, insomnia, and stressors. You want the sense that all is well, even in the worst of times. The brain develops thought patterns, the more you focus on empowering thoughts for falling asleep, the more easily you'll be able to revisit these thoughts in your future driftings.

Touching Back on Visualizing

One powerful technique that we'll close out this section discussing is vividly visualizing. As interesting as it sounds, this has become the most powerful way I can "think myself to sleep." Think of shows like Rick and Morty, and movies like The Matrix or Fear and Loathing in Las Vegas, where the reality is bending, colors are changing. When I am able to see the frames of unique, strange, vivid pictures, or simply go back to a memory of a strange dream, I have found this to be one of the most powerful ways to direct my "thinking", and quickly doze off.

I think you'll find it incredibly effective.

D. Body Position and Movement

The majority of people are side sleepers. Less are back sleepers and still fewer are stomach sleepers. Ultimately you should do what allows you the most comfort to sleep. But also know that you can train yourself to sleep in a different position with some consistent practice and discipline.

From a health perspective, back and side sleeping are most optimal. Stomach sleeping can be quite problematic to breathing and overall posture, but sometimes that's just the way it works.

I used to sleep much more on my side, but over the years, sharing my bed I've found it much more comfortable to sleep like a corpse. I find my body, back and overall circulation flows the best when I drift to sleep while on my back.

From the discussions on trauma I will say that if you're feeling particularly riled up while trying to drift to sleep, you can place your hands on your waist, stomach or heart. By resting your hands on your body you create containment and a feeling of ease.

If I'm particularly anxious when falling asleep, I will place my hands on my heart. This is one of the greatest hacks I've found for creating a sense of safety and allowing myself to fall asleep. But I've noticed that circulation in my forearms and hands will become limited from my bent elbows. You'll have to play with this and see what works best for you, if it's worth the trade off.

The other thing to consider is a weight-blanket. We'll discuss this more in the section on accessories in part 11.

7. PRIMING THE BODY

As a human, you're naturally encoded to sleep well. If you "live well", and hack ways to be more ancestrally consistent with how we lived for millions of years, you will naturally sleep better. You by no means need to do all of these, but they will help you.

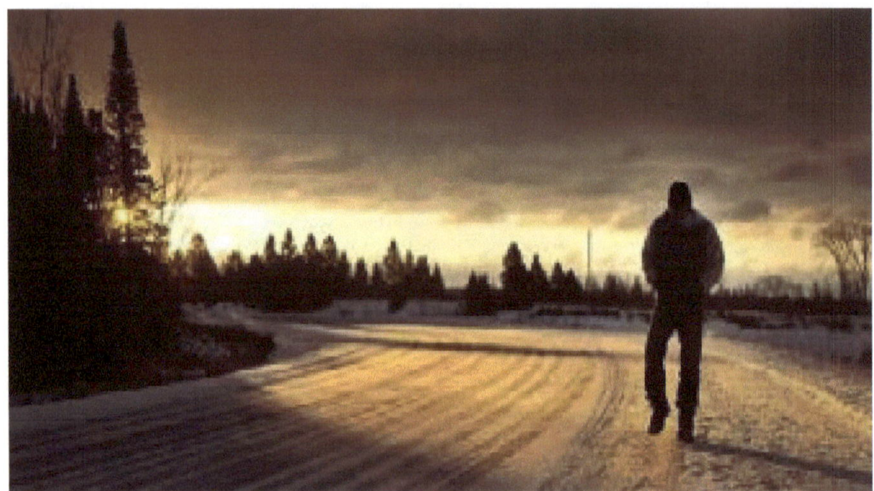

Image: https://krixluther.com/benefits-of-morning-walk/

I. Get Outside

Modern humans have lost touch with nature. One of the very first things we ancestrally experienced waking up was direct light from the sky. Daylight more directly reaching our eyes and skin triggers our body's natural clock. It helps signal your natural body clock cycle that the day has officially begun. When your body experiences signals such as this early in the day, it then is better set to wind down in the evening and naturally drift to sleep.

II. Move

Get physical movement early in the day, preferably outdoors. Ancestrally we humans often walked for miles daily, tracking, hunting, sprinting. Now many of us are rarely this active even monthly. A morning walk can be a powerful 1-2 knockout activity. In fact, an outdoor walk has become one of the most potent recovery and refreshing modalities I've personally found.

You don't have to be a gym rat or extreme athlete to benefit from this, but getting a healthy dose of physical activity daily (even if it's just a brief walk), will play a role in improving sleep quality. Not only that, but there's a whole slew of other health benefits with movement and exercise.[25]

III. Experience Sunlight

The sun is a powerful star that provides an incredible amount of energy and life for our planet. Humans evolved to experience sunlight directly. I've written and recorded several videos and posts dedicated entirely to this topic and the importance of this nutrient. Here we touch briefly, and specifically, on how it impacts sleep.

There are tremendous benefits to sunlight exposure.[26] Skin doctors have been trained to protect the skin from sun at all costs, even if it means wrecking health in other areas. Proverbially they have thrown the baby out with the bathwater when looking at how sunlight impacts overall human health. In fact, doctors have classified UV from the planet's sky as carcinogenic! [27] Unfortunately they are zeroing in on melanoma and the burning / aging effects UV radiation may have, without taking into account everything else the body gains from this powerful nutrient.

Do we really think natural chronic sun exposure is carcinogenic in healthy amounts? Humans evolved outside for millions of years.

Without restating all the information I've discussed on light - letting a healthy dose (not burning, but being outside daily 30-60 minutes) of sunlight every single day reach your skin actually does more good than harm for your overall health and will improve your sleep quality. In fact, some studies even show it reduces your overall risk of skin cancer. [..]

Get sunlight, its benefits are far reaching and risks are far outweighed by its cons.

IV. Ground

Our bodies are electrical systems. The electron-transport chain is the primary way our cells generate ATP (their energy). Our heart runs on electrical impulses. Our brain neurons fire electrical signals. Ancestrally we slept on surfaces much more closely connected to the earth and grounding force.

Ground is an electrical term that relates to when you are able to connect to a solid source of earth ground to neutralize and send back excess electrical build-up. By grounding, it allows the surplus charge and electrical energy that can build up to be neutralized and sent back to the earth rather than built up. Walking barefoot on earth, even for 5 mins can greatly improve this.

IV. Heat Exposure

Although you don't want heat during sleep, any sort of heat exposure during your day: sauna, bath or shower, can aid in detoxification, relaxation and fluid flow. It helps in detoxification through sweat and also flushes fluid to improve circulation. Overall this also acts as a hermetic, environmental stressor when done in healthy amounts to enhance overall vitality and sleep quality. Numerous studies have been done to show the health benefits of sauna and regular sweating and how it improves overall health. [..]

V. Cold Exposure

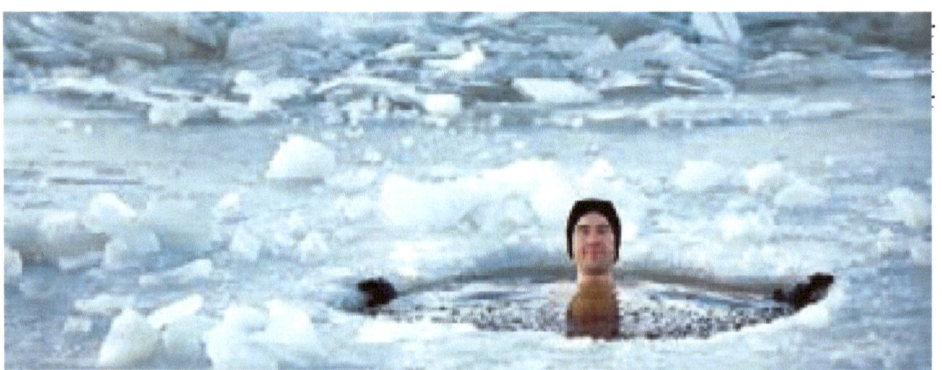

Image: https://www.peakendurancesport.com/other/pouring-cold-water-on-ice-baths/

That said, cold exposure is something our ancestors likely experienced regularly, and it shows some serious health benefits. [28] Exposing your body to cold exposure will improve deep sleep significantly. It will also trigger glutathione (a potent antioxidant) production in the body naturally.

I have built my own chest freezer cold plunge on my deck. I used to go to a local facility in Austin that gave me access to a sauna, followed by a cold and hot plunge in water that is 49F -> 107F. I cycled back and forth in the process. I now usually do the cold plunge up to my neck for 5 minutes 1-2 times per session, 3-4 days / week and directly notice deeper, longer sleep. Submerging my entire head in for 15-20 seconds each time I jump into the plunge refreshes my whole body.

Cryotherapy using cold water seems to show better recovery results for most, but the evidence isn't entirely conclusive. It certainly seems like crossing icy streams and lakes of cold waters fed by glaciers and cold rivers are more ancestrally consistent than encountering air below -170F shirtless for 3-4 minutes. In either case, the point is, cold exposure is powerful at improving sleep. 29]

For many, this may not be easily accessible, but one can still take cold showers and take cold baths from time to time. For cold baths, just empty out that freezer ice maker in a bath of the coldest water, even in Texas it will get a colder (~ 55F plunge) which is enough to trigger many of the benefits. As much as I hate the initial shock of the ice cold water on my body, the effects and benefits are clear.

Consider cold water immersion if you're consistently struggling with deep sleep.

If you're a chronic light sleeper, feel like you're seriously lacking recovery and deep sleep, I can't recommend cold water immersion strongly enough. Showers (at least 60 secs) will help, but cold plunges and baths will have a greater order of magnitude and improvement due to the colder impact.

8. SLEEP ENVIRONMENT FUNDAMENTALS

Let's talk about the environment your body experiences and where you sleep. When we think of the environment, we think of the area outside our bodies, but it also turns out, inside our gut is another environment we also have, we just don't see it.

"*It also turns out inside our gut is another environment* ***we also have***, *we just don't see it.*"

We'll talk briefly about both because they both matter.

Internal Environment

What do you expose the inside of your body to? Is it a concoction of triggering foods, stimulants, and alcohol, inflaming, triggering molecules, or is it actually being treated with love and care that supports the intricate and sensitive system it is?

I wrote a book on diet The Carnivore Diet. If you experience anxiety, gut issues, skin issues, autoimmune, inflammation, even sleep, your diet could be a MAJOR variable.

The human gut is a very thin, single-cell junction layer, and many compounds can penetrate it. This leads to a whole slew of problems and issues from triggering autoimmune reactions to higher levels of inflammation, to anxiety, you name it. Considering and adjusting your diet is one of the most powerful things you can do to support your health, vitality, and overall cognitive and physical performance.

Coffee / Stimulants

Let's talk about caffeine. It works by plugging the body's adenosine receptors. Normally adenosine would build up in these receptors as the day progresses, slowly creating "sleep pressure" as the day progresses. By fitting caffeine into these receptors, it blocks adenosine from building up and creates the effect of being highly alert often at the cost of inhibiting our natural sleepiness needed at the end of our day.

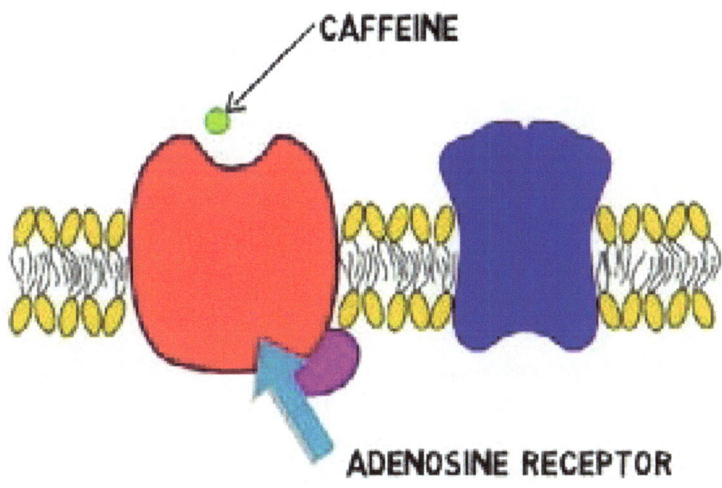

Image source: Neuroscientifically Challenged

Caffeine has a half-life of 6-12 hours (see below figure). That means, depending on your body type, an 8oz mug of 120mg caffeine in coffee at noon will still be a 65mg caffeine dose in your body 12 hours later by midnight. That's not a good thing for sleep. Some people can metabolize it faster, but even if you do, it's still hard to become caffeine-free even in 24 hours. It just stays too long in the system.

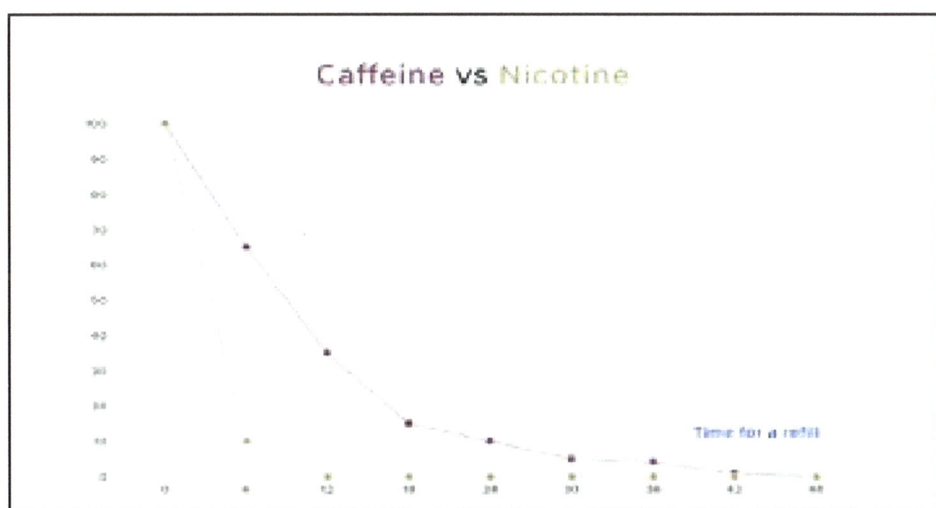

Image: Comparison caffeine vs nicotine half-life

Coffee comes with a slew of other concerns. Polyphenols can be harmful, leading to leaky gut and damaged DNA [30]. The antioxidative benefits are parrotted by the big coffee industry, but the reality is the majority of coffee beans, and coffee consumed even in its best form, is often contaminated with pesticides and mold toxins that also may lead to poor health. Although the amounts vary, and many will claim these toxins are everywhere, - I believe we can mitigate them by avoiding high offending foods such as most coffees. Be careful. [31]

Personally, my metabolism of coffee is normal, but after learning about the quality and potential negative effects, I decided to quit coffee. I had been a daily java lover for nearly a half-decade. I was totally hooked. Hooked on the flavor, the morning jolt, the helping of passing my morning #2's. I just really enjoyed coffee all around. But I knew it was impacting my sleep quality and was creating a bit of anxiety during my day.

Day 1 Quitting my coffee cold turkey, I was hurting. Feeling lethargic, foggy, and experiencing withdrawal headaches.
Day 2 Was more of the same.
Day 3 I was wondering if this would ever get better.
Day 5 After almost a week, I felt like a totally different person.

The first night I slept without coffee I woke up the next day feeling like I had slept deeper than I could ever recall. It was a deeper feeling of restedness, and that persisted even more so through those initial 3-5 days transitioning off the coffee addiction.

I've been coffee/caffeine-free since Christmas 2018. I've yet to have a desire to limit my sleep quality and can count on one hand the # of times I've had a decaf / caffeinated espresso/coffee by chance. Another major impact I've noticed with caffeine is the duration of my REM sleep.

I've spoken to a number of clients and friends about this. Caffeine directly lowers REM in almost everyone I know who tracks their REM stage using an Oura Ring. This, in effect, directly impacts how rested you feel the next day mentally. Remember, REM is a critical stage of sleep where we store and file learning, memories and clear our mental cognitive abilities for the next day. With coffee, I've seen REM consistently drop by as much as 80% in people. It's a vicious cycle that keeps you trapped, feeling the need for it - even more so - the next day.

Nicotine

Opt for natural and organic alternatives that have a much shorter half-life, but that can still deliver a punch and oomphf to get you going in daily lulls. Personally, I really enjoy Nicotine, and there's a number of individuals who promote it as a powerful performance enhancer. I hate the idea of smoking or vaping.

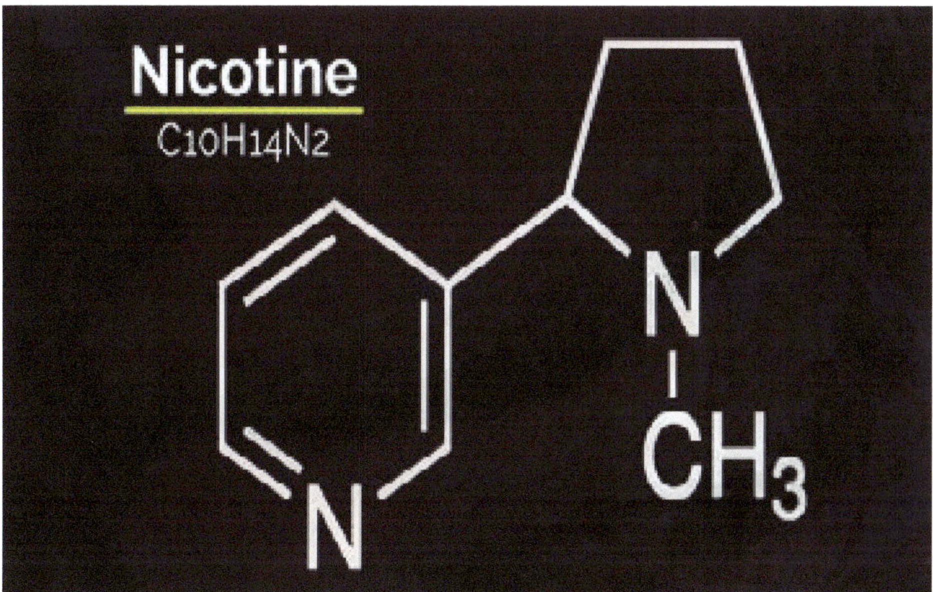

Vaping

I've tried a variety of vaping devices: Smoks and Juuls (only 3% tobacco flavor). I enjoyed the act of inhaling and the nicotine it gave me, but I consistently noticed throat issues and swelling of my lymph nodes from the inhaling of the chemicals. To me, it was a sign these devices were causing inflammation, hurting my respiratory system and were unsustainable for my body.

The delivery of Nicotine is tricky. As I don't prefer smoking, I tried lozenges and gums from companies like Nicorette, but have since backed off as they are loaded with other chemicals and are unnatural.

Snus

I was finally turned on to snus by my buddy Kyle Kingsbury [..] when we spent a weekend hunting together. He's a big plant medicine guy (psilocybin, ayahuasca, nicotine, mushrooms for performance - his podcast brings depth to these topics), and he taught me a tremendous amount. On that weekend, we were hunting, and his snus became a comrade I'm glad I paired with. Since then, I've found organic natural forms of tobacco that I very much enjoy, but which I taper off towards the end of my evenings. I don't notice a negative impact on my sleep quality in the same way as caffeine.

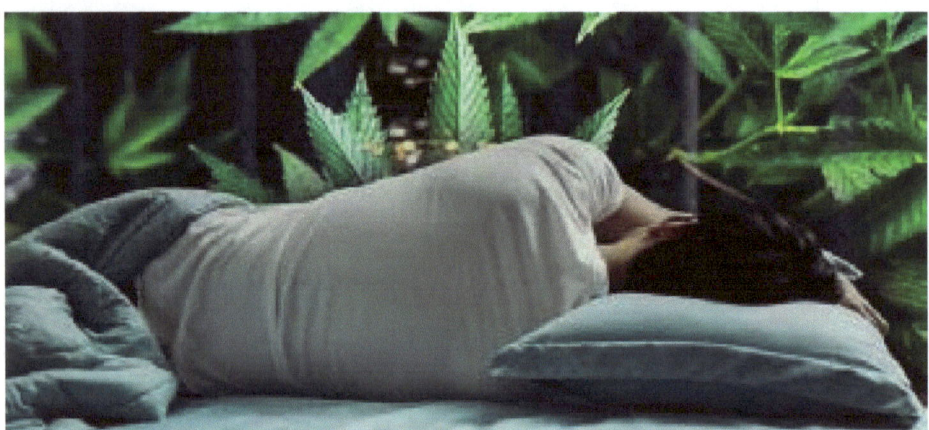

Marijuana

What about Marijuana? Many consider CBD and THC as excellent vehicles to improve their sleep. But here's the thing, their mechanisms actually negatively impact sleep quality. [32]

If you've ever fallen asleep to a powerful Indica strain of marijuana, you'll know the body's relaxation and drowsiness are profound, and you easily drift off. But most people won't dream when they sleep on weed. This is because the cannabinoids suppress the REM cycle.

When cannabis users stop smoking, they often experience vivid and intense dreams. This is because those who regularly smoke marijuana - especially when falling asleep, prevent their minds from experiencing the valuable full REM stages allowing them to process dreams regularly. That build-up comes out in those moments of no marijuana. Dr. Matthew Walker, a renowned sleep researcher, discusses this in this interview (NSFW, some language) with Joe Rogan how marijuana, as well as alcohol, can impact sleep.

Keep this in mind, and consider the consequences, that sleep you think you may be getting from these substances may actually be confused with sedation, which is not truly sleeping.

Alcohol

With all these substances, people react differently. Different alcohols impact individuals in different ways. Tequila will often give energy to many, while Vodka can be more sedative. Though all alcohol is considered a depressant, some simply impact individuals differently.

Alcohol suppresses REM sleep and lowers overall stages of quality sleep. In fact, one common note for alcoholics coming off booze is experiencing symptoms of delirium tremens. This can happen to a degree where the individuals will even experience hallucination-like visions. Researchers believe this may be due to the build-up of REM cycle pressure the brain is attempting to relieve while taking the individual into dreams to process this even when they are "awake."

Needless to say, both drinking and smoking damages our bodies in many ways and does not support optimal sleep. If you're going to do either, try to limit the days you do; engage earlier in the day, limit consumption and hydrate and physically move later in your day to help metabolize and return your body closer to baseline prior to sleeping.

Cutting out long half-life stimulants and psychoactive substances such as alcohol and cannabis can have a major impact on the quality and ability to fall asleep.

Let's shift gears and talk about what's outside the digestive system of your body.

9. External Environment

Temperature

Our ancestors likely slept in colder temperatures, impacted more by the environment. When the body cools, it tends to fall asleep better. By reducing the temperature, you will assist both in falling asleep easier and sleeping deeper.

If possible, get a programmable thermostat that can gradually lower the temperature of your sleeping room down all throughout the night, to a lcool temperature that mirrors what the outdoors would do. By gradually reducing the temperature, and then warming back up, you will use temperature to regulate and guide you through optimal sleep.

Here's how my NEST thermostat schedule looks:

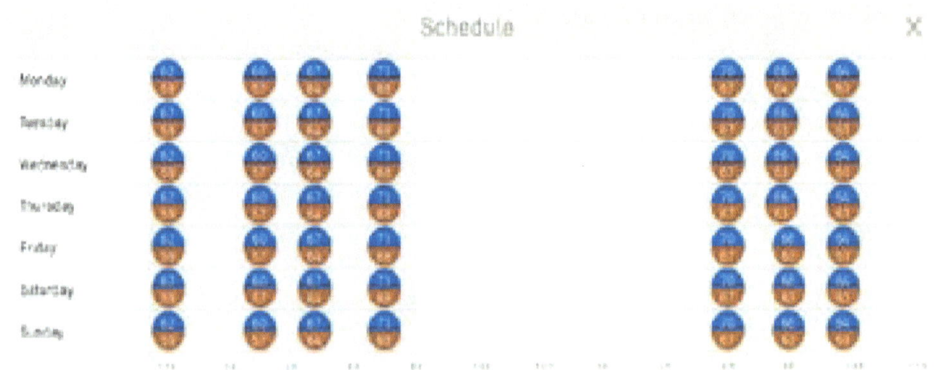

Pre Industrial Society Sleep Schedules

In one of the most comprehensive sleep studies [33] of preindustrial societies, I found researchers concluded that temperature was likely as powerful a regulator of sleep as light.

In this study published in CELL, researchers observed three equatorial preindustrial societies and found that:

1. Sleep onset occurred on average 3.3 hrs after sunset.
2. Waking occurred approximately 1hr before sunrise.
3. In the summer tribes slept an hour less.
4. Napping, in the traditional sense, was rare, but resting was common.

Sleep Surface Temp

The other thing I actively do is cool the sleep surface I sleep on. Ancestrally we slept on the ground and cooler things. ChiliPad (full disclosure - I am an affiliate) has made a water cooled device that allows the surface of your mattress to stay cool. This allows for a couple of things: 1) It cools the surface of the bed - I tend to sleep hot 2) It allows me to use a big winter heavyweight comforter blanket which weighs down on me without my body getting too hot at night. This creates a feeling of safety and comfort I previously could not experience because the bed would get too hot.

If you're interested in learning more about this, I created a full review of the ChiliPad and compared it to its predecessor, the Ooler Sleep System here. In the video description I also provide a discount code if interested.

This combination of being able to stay cool, while using a heavy blanket, has really upped my feeling of safety and ease. As I discussed in the mental aspect of sleep, I have personally noticed a profound impact on the quality of my sleep based on the emotional state I'm in. This has been further substantiated by the trauma studies and literature I've studied in particular with Peter A. Levine.

Light in Bedroom

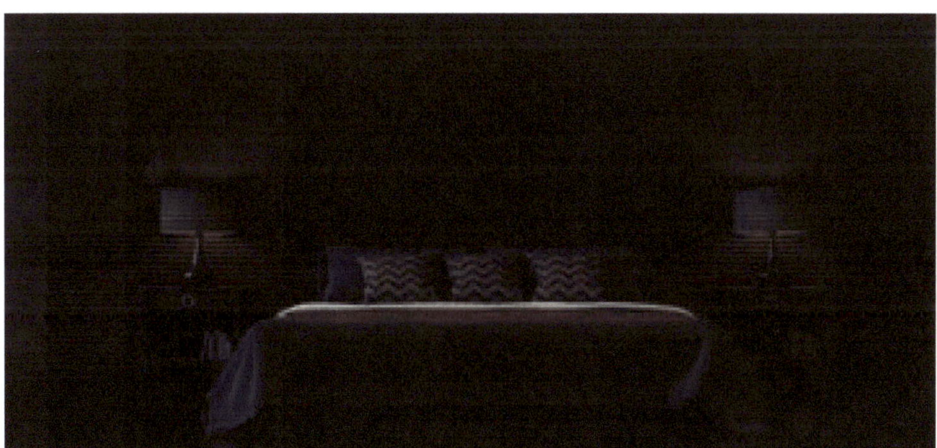

Image source: https://www.smartnora.com/blogs/nora-blogs/dark-bedroom-better-sleep

This nutrient, yes that's right I said it, "nutrient," is so important. Did you know your skin cells have light receptors on them? Artificial light hitting your skin can impact the circadian rhythm and the body's ability to produce hormones and fully drop into sleep [34].

Weight gain and disease are also being shown with light exposure during sleep. [35] You really don't want your body exposed to light while sleeping.

With respect to sleep, you must make the room dark to the point that your low light adjusted eyes cannot see your hands in front of your face. The amount of light generated from street lights, buildings, and artificial light sources in a house can be substantially more intense than the moon and stars hundreds of thousands of miles away.

Artificial blue light has barely been around for 150 years. Before that mankind mostly experienced fire and some form of red hues for 100's of thousands of years. Depending on who you talk with, anthropologists say fire was discovered between 1.2M - 200,000 years ago. In either case, that's a huge discrepancy in comparison to artificial light. The length of time we've had to evolve biologically to adapt to this new light after sundown is literally non-existent. And it's making a major impact on society's sleep hygiene. Consider blue blocker glasses at night after sunset and consider changing out blue bulbs in your home for red bulbs.

I found blackout blinds from Bed Bath and Beyond that work exceptionally well and are relatively inexpensive (shopped around Amazon, Google Shopping), $200-$300 to completely blackout my loft. Get a solid handyman who can install a dowel (think of how your closet hangers sit) across the top of your window/wall and get that area blacked out. There's something powerful about sleeping in total darkness that our bodies experience that allows them to feel safe and drift even deeper into sleep.

nnEMF

Non native electromagnetic frequencies are waves of radiation we don't see that are not natural to the ancestral environment for humans. Things like cell signals, Wifi and Bluetooth are just a few examples of nnEMF. These can have a powerful impact on sleep quality. Unplug and turn off everything in your room. Use black electrical tape to cover any LEDs and light sources that are plugged in that you keep near your sleeping area. Sleeping your laptop often still leaves on WiFi and Bluetooth, so shut it down at night.

If you use your phone as an alarm, which I do myself, make sure it's in airplane mode and purchase an EMF sleeve that will shield it's radiation and slip your phone into that at night. Even airplane modes can release EMF.

Sound and Noise

I'm a city slicker, and I've lived in cities for the majority of my adult life. Manhattan, Seattle, and now Austin. I like the convenience and living of being able to walk and bicycle to get around, but I hate the light and noise at night.

As a result of this, I've now specifically chosen apartments that face away from noise locations (roads, shops, bars, etc.) and have better acoustics for noise prevention built into their units.

I think white noise machines are great, as they help us sleep with some vibration and noise - that way we're not totally destroyed in other noisy travel sleep situations. My ChiliPad makes a low-level hum sound when running at night, which serves as a great white noise machine. But you don't need a ChiliPad to get white noise. There are apps on phones and devices for ~ $20 online that can serve to make a light wind/white noise hum.

After living in Manhattan and Seattle on busy streets, even with my white noise machines, I found that the street noise could startle me from time to time. As a result, and wanting to be more adapted to traveling in other sleep environments and not feel anxious, I started using earplugs. This took me a long time (several months) to finally get used to, but now I am extremely comfortable using plugs and prefer them even in an extremely quiet environment.

"One of the biggest parts of sleep is the mental aspect of it"

As I mentioned in the beginning section of this book, one of the biggest parts of sleep is the mental aspect of it. If you're constantly worried, on edge, or anxious about your sleeping situation, why not build in habits to better handle and deal with them? By always using a mask and earplugs, I can sleep almost anywhere, anytime, without the concerns of being startled in some unexpected way, especially in a room or sleep situation that's less than ideal. I find this greatly alleviates anxiety around the darkness, and sound situation of a hotel room or Airbnb. If it's a consistent sleep location that is within my control, I look for ways to enhance darkness, coolness, and quietness in addition to using these things. This is the eye mask I prefer.

Bed

Of course, no sleep environment discussion would be complete without discussing what bed you're using. You will spend 1/3 of your life on this piece of furniture, and it will make a sizable impact on your ability to sleep.

I've invested $1,000s in different types of beds. I've tested ultra firm, ultra plush, and everything in between. In fact, my last experience buying a mattress from Macy's involved returning one that was too firm, one that was too soft and landing on a final one that was in the middle, just perfect. Each mattress I slept on for 60-90 days before exchanging in with their restocking option.

The type of bed you decide to buy will likely come down to a combination of personal preference, to how you feel when lying on the mattress, and your budget. Personally, I prefer to go to a mattress store so that I can talk with a salesperson and physically lay down on the mattresses I'm considering for purchase. I'm not a fan of buying a bed you've never tried.

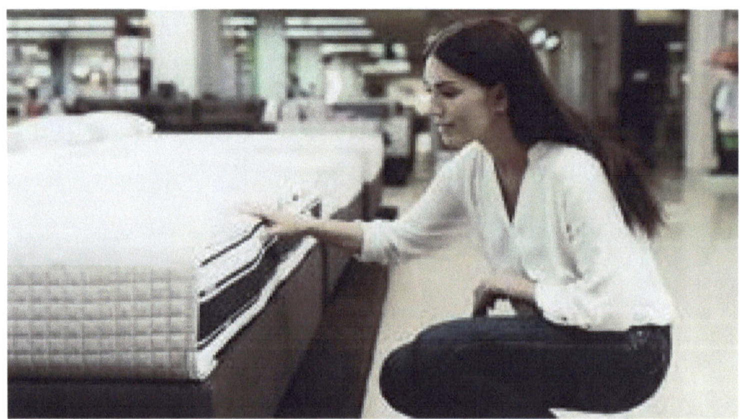

In store buying tips:

- Find a professional salesperson who has experience and knows what they are talking about. If you get a sense, they are new and/or just don't provide the feedback you want, ask for input from another.
- Determine your budget. This will help the salesperson determine the class and your best options.
- Share your sleep preferences and positions, are you a back-sleeper, side-sleeper, stomach sleeper, do you run hot, cold or fairly neutral?
- Do you want a soft mattress, or do you prefer it much more firm?
- How long do you intend to keep the mattress?

Keep in mind beds and their softness will depend on how long they've been on the store floor and how old they are. Ask the rep about the history of the floor models so you can gauge how well it'll compare to your brand new purchase of the floor sample. There will be a break-in period for the average person of 45-60 days.

All these questions will give the salesperson a sense of what is most optimal for you. Mattresses can range from $300 - $10,000. You want to utilize your budget to best meet your needs. You wouldn't want to invest 75% of your budget into durability if you intend on moving in 12-24 months, won't bring that bed with you.

Material can improve support, coolness, and longevity, but often adds substantially to the initial costs. Sleeping position and preference of feel are also big factors to consider, arguably some of the biggest. Side sleepers will need more softness. Firm mattresses (popular in many Asian cultures) are typically better for heavier, larger back sleepers.

My first purchase when I moved to Austin was an extremely firm mattress, and as much as I would love it, I kept waking up in the middle of the night. It was an ultra-firm that I thought would be perfect for my back-sleeping self. After weeks of leaving my safe on the bed in different parts to soften it up, I still could not sleep soundly all through the night. Ultimately I returned it and ended up overcorrecting to a too-soft mattress.

Back Pain

You may feel a bit of soreness when you wake up, but if it persists beyond 5-10 mins, then you may be lacking proper support. Support comes with the quality of the spring structure and materials used in making the mattress. One reason I prefer spending more on my bed vs. getting something lower cost when I have the money, is exactly to get proper support. Lower quality beds will experience failing springs and "taco" and lead to back pain and improper sleep support.

9. WHEN SHOULD YOU SLEEP

Sigh one of the single most challenging things for most of us.

When you go to bed will impact the quality of your sleep. Deep sleep is most experienced during the beginning stages of our sleep. REM is experienced more towards the end of core sleep, right before waking. If you go to sleep later than usual, you'll notice deep sleep gets, and thus physical recovery suffering. If you have an early wake-up call, REM cycles are limited and mental and cognitive experiences are more impacted. This is why waking up early can be so difficult mentally and emotionally. And this is why elite athletes like Lebron James, Tom Brady, and Roger Federer are all known to sleep early and exceptionally long.

I used to think this was a one-size-fits-all, and there is an optimal sleep schedule for humans universally. Through working with people and seeing consistent patterns and habits, I've come to realize it's not always the case. Sleep schedules may be genetically coded in our biology, and variation may have been advantageous to our species' survival.

Let's take a look at what sleeping on an ancestral schedule for preindustrial equatorial tribes from three distinct parts of the world [33] looks like. In this study, researchers found:

1. Duration 5.7-7.1 hrs / night.
2. Winter sleep duration increased by 56 mins.
3. Sleep time was 3.3 hours after sunset.
4. Awakening occurred 1 hour prior to sunrise.
5. Napping and insomnia were both very limited.
6. Temperature seemed to be a primary factor in sleep.

A few things to consider when interpreting this data: 1) These are pre-industrial tribes 2) They live more closely to the equator than most of us 3) They sleep outside in a "camping" like environment. 4) Lastly, they get lots of daily physical movement and sunlight.

That said, if we adjust this to say a 6:00 am sunrise and a 6:00 pm sunset for most locations and try and average things out we could say that an optimal sleeping schedule would be:

a. Going to be in bed between 9:00-10:00 pm
b. Waking up around 5:00 am
c. Increasing sleep duration in winter
d. Decreasing sleep duration in summer

I'm not here to tell you to end your social life.

Of course, I realize this isn't always socially optimal. I'm not here to tell you to end your social life. I'm simply here to help you best understand and optimize the consistency and quality of your sleep and recovery. For most people, this schedule will support a more consistent, high-quality sleep routine.

Our bodies run on a rhythm called the circadian. Approximately every 24 hours we have high and low energy phases our body naturally cycles through. We naturally experience shifts and adjustments of energy and vitality based on our clock. Depending on your genetic chronotype, you may be more of an "early bird" or "night owl." Also, depending on your age and life phase, you can shift into different types. Teenagers are wolves that stay up late and sleep late. Older adults tend to be early birds sleeping and rising early.

Chronotypes

Chronotypes are a typing coined by certain sleep psychologists for categorizing different sleep schedules. The first time I heard of Chronotypes, I was skeptical. After doing a bit of digging, I've found them quite interesting, and this may be worth looking into further if you struggle to get to bed early.

According to Dr. Michael Breus and his great book, The Power of When he defines four distinct Chronotypes: Dolphin, Lion, Bear and Wolf. Each type is named after the animal, which most similarly represents that sleep/wake pattern.

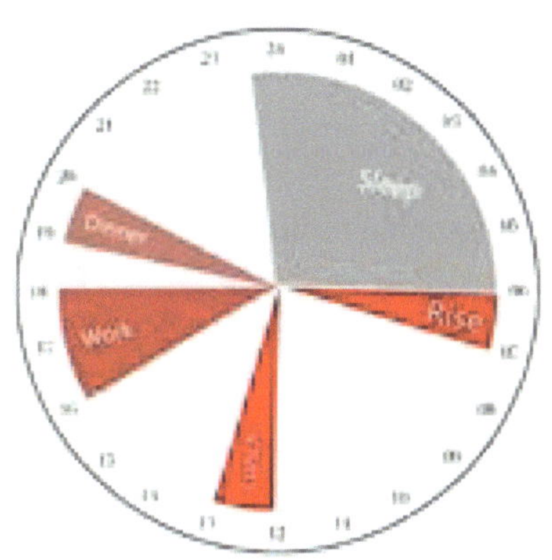

Dolphins

Dolphins sleep hemispherically. Only one side of the brain is ever sleeping, as they must constantly swim and stay moving to avoid drowning and dying. Human "dolphins" tend to be more neurotic and impulsive. They can often be tired and wired with nervous energy. They are the insomniacs, the individuals who struggle to sleep. They rarely sleep more than 6 core hours. They will wake and snooze at 6-7am, may skip breakfast, eat lunch 12-1pm, have peak alertness 4-6pm, 7-8pm have dinner. 11:30pm attempt to sleep for the evening.

Lions

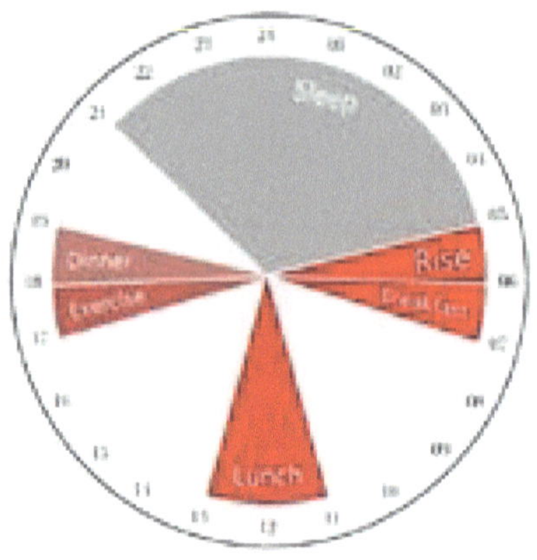

In the wild, lions often rise before dawn, hunt and feed at dawn. Lion chronotypes hit the ancestral alignment lottery for their circadian rhythm. They are the people who are early risers and early to bed. They are often the achievers who make the most of their days. Their energy levels and mood peak in the morning and steadily decline throughout the day.

They typically rise 5-6am, eat an early, hearty breakfast 6-7am and then attack the day. They'll have a sizable lunch 11-1pm and then a very light dinner before drifting to bed 9-10pm. Exercising in the early evening can give them a boost of energy, as their evenings are usually lower energy.

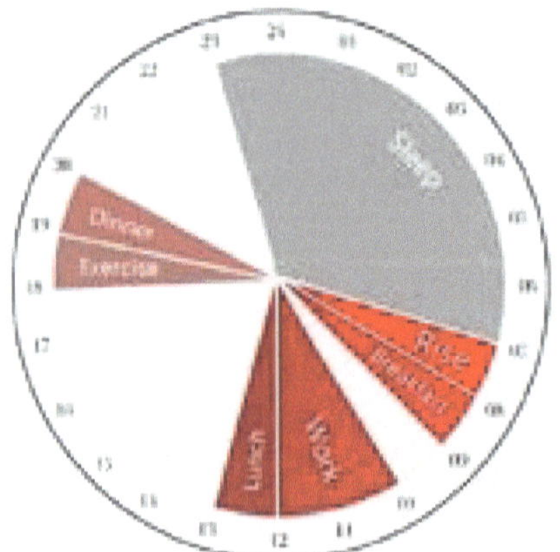

Bears

Bear chronotypes encompass the majority of people. They are the doers of the world that make it go round. They typically wake at sunrise about 7am, breakfast 8-9 am, start waking up by 10am-12pm to do work for their day. 12-1pm they partake in lunch. Exercising at 6pm and then having dinner 7-8pm is optimal. 11-12pm is when they start winding down for bed.

Wolves

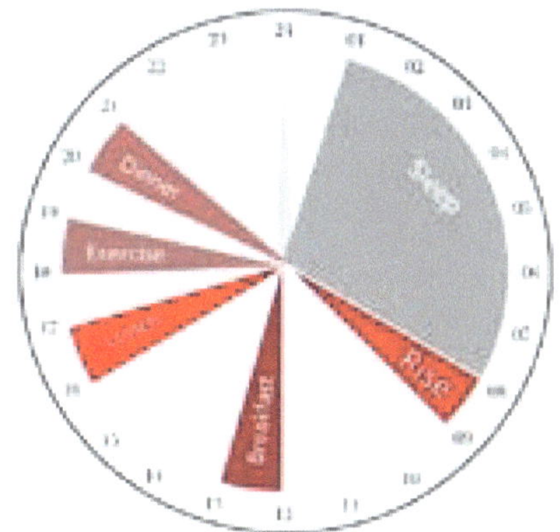

Wolf chronotypes are the latter-day patterned folks. They struggle to wake up before 8am. They aren't hungry in the morning and struggle to feel clear-headed until 11am. By 1pm they are hungry and eat their "breakfast." They feel an energy dip post lunch, but then feel a surge of energy from 4-7pm. They typically exercise 6-7pm. They prefer to eat a later dinner at 8-9pm. They start to wind down around 12am, but frequently don't fall asleep until after 1am.

Do any of these habits/patterns sound like you? I found myself falling into one, in particular, most of the time. No one is better than another, though arguably for longevity and optimal productivity, lions appear to take the cake. They have a circadian rhythm that aligns with daytime activities most optimally and seem to support optimal hormone, sleep, and productivity.

Ultimately, when you decide to sleep and wake, has to work best for your life. I share this to give you an understanding. Although some claim this is genetic, from what we've seen in pre-industrial societies and other data gathered, the majority of us are going to sleep with light and temperature as the most influential moderators. I find that I'm mostly a lion, but can drift into a bear. My deep sleep is almost always reduced if I stay up much beyond 10:30pm.

10. SLEEP PREPARATION

Everything we've discussed ultimately leads to optimal sleep "preparation." But in this section, I want to go into the specifics of what we're "doing" to prepare before going to bed in the evening.

As we've learned, light and temperature are big signalers for the body. As your bedtime approaches, for you to be optimizing for light and temperature, the biggest levers are:

Evening Lighting

As the sun sets, light spectrums shift more towards red and away from ultraviolet, violet, and green. Humans discovered fire anywhere from 200,000 years to 1.7M years [illegible]

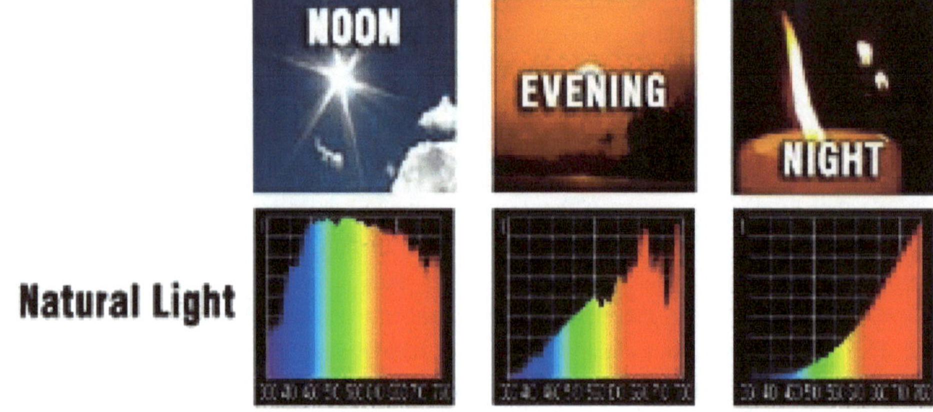

Image Source: https://www.sunlightinside.com/light-and-health/comparing-philips-hue-natural-light/

Remove blue and green spectrums of light. Personally, I utilize smart bulbs where I can control the color, and change my lighting to match hues of the outdoors, ultimately post-sunset, only red hues close to the color of fire. Blue blockers are a valuable tool to enhance this further, as we're often limited in controlling lighting on our screens (tvs, laptops, iPads, phones) or in restaurants and other establishments.

Full disclosure: I'm a big fan of RaOptics: https://raoptics.com/collections/glasses. Founder Matt Maruca has done an excellent job making lenses that specifically block these frequencies of light, while sitting in stylish frames you can wear out. Use code "karnivore" at checkout for 10% off if you decide to pick up a pair.

Either way, make an effort to limit blue and red spectrums from hitting your retina and suprachiasmatic nucleus in the evening. By limiting exposure to blue and green light spectrums after sunset, you will be avoiding the confusing signal being sent to the human that the sun is still up.

"Our bodies did not evolve to experience the volume and intensity of artificial blue / green light we now have in society late into our evenings."

Our bodies did not evolve to experience the volume and intensity of artificial blue / green light we now have in society late into our evenings. Remember, we evolved with the stars and fire over the last several hundreds of thousands of years. Thomas Edison invented the light bulb 150 years ago. These spectrums confuse our biology and suppress its ability to produce sleep onset signals and sleep naturally much deeper.

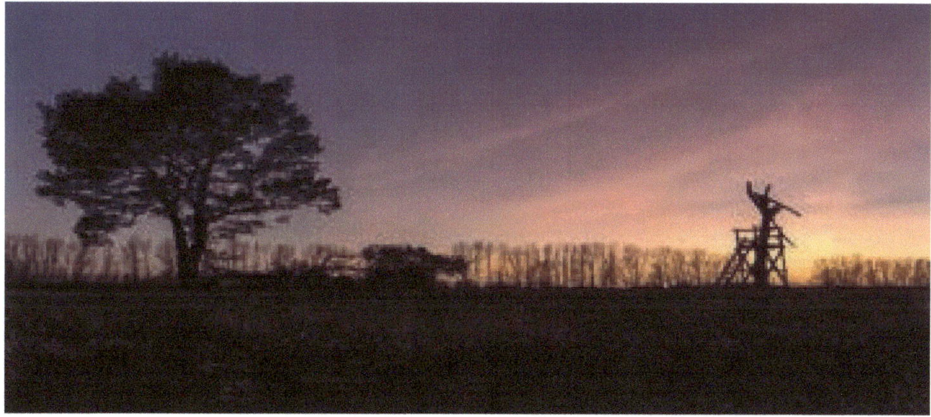

Dusk Lighting

Heading into spring and summer, I've been experimenting with using very dim red lights and completely avoiding large screens such as TVs and laptops after sunset. The sun is setting around 8 now, and I simply don't turn any lights on after dusk. (Except a 10-watt red bulb in the master bathroom to see when making final preparations right before sleep.)

Depending on your home's window situation, this may not be practical. But I have noticed a significant increase in sleep pressure, quality, and ability to easily fall asleep quickly compared with watching TV, or staring at a computer screen and having even moderate amounts of red lights on after dusk.

When I do this, I am yawning quite strongly within 90 minutes after sunset.

During the 90 minutes after sunset, activities I have found quite rewarding and can still be done include:

- Listening to an audiobook/podcast
- Streaming show at minimal brightness off my iPhone (smaller screen)
- Stretching and foam rolling to release body tension

In cases where I MUST be on my computer or larger screen, I will turn the brightness settings all the way down. I'll also dial in the f.lux setting to a very red hue, night mode, to contrast text as white against darker backgrounds. I make sure I am wearing a pair of blue blocker glasses.

Evening Activity

It seems fairly obvious to me, but if you're going for late night sprints or heavy lifts, you're dialing up, not down, our physiology. This will negatively impact your ability to relax and drift into sleep if done too closely to bedtime. Restrain from extraneous exercise at least 3 hours prior to bedtime. This activates the nervous system, and when we don't give it enough time, it does not settle to a level to support easily drifting into sleep

Ironically an evening walk at a moderate, **NOT elevated pace** has been shown to be calming, meditative, and supports digestion and higher sleep quality.[37]

When my anxiety and depression were at their peak, I wanted to control everything. Just about anything outside of a very tight regimen would tip me over. Being able to sleep well was nearly impossible unless I stuck to a very regimented plan. But having such a dependent mindset on the rigidity of that routine created anxiety on sleeping outside my routine. It also played havoc on my social life flexibility. I still like to have a routine, but with the work on my mindset and practices around diet, lifestyle, and priming my body for optimal functioning, I no longer have to follow such a strict regimen to guarantee quality sleep. I've worked on calming and supporting the foundation of my sleep through all the things in this book.

The Last Meal

Eating a lighter meal, three plus hours prior to sleep, will greatly improve your sleep quality. I haven't entirely pieced together exactly what the ancestral consistency is here, but eating after sunset has been studied, and there's plenty of evidence to support the negative health consequences. [38] [39] [40] Our bodies seem to have evolved to eating more earlier in our days, and it is reflected in how we metabolize and respond to food with hormones.

I continually scratch my head, observing people who eat after 8, 9 or later at night. It's a total sabotage of your hormones and your body's capacity to sleep optimally. This is a HARD rule I have made for myself for almost 10 years now, and I've stayed true to it. Unless you're in a state of severe nutrient deficiency, the health benefits and overall optimization will be highly supported by eating earlier.

With the The Power of When quiz you can determine your chronotype. This may help you learn more about your preferred sleep timing. Even with a "chronotype" that shows you as a late-night person, most science is strong that earlier sleep will optimize even those night "wolves." It's hard to stay up light when screens and artificial light are cut. 95% of cases the science is real - you are much better to avoid that late-night snacking and limit food consumption after sundown.

Sorry evening socialites, but evening eating is actually quite damaging to your hormones, long term health and in particular, your sleep quality! If you want to be optimized, this could be a huge health variable to consider shifting. And I'm not here to destroy social lives, but if you're really struggling with sleep issues, strict discipline to get back on track and build momentum may be worth the temporary sacrifice.

In fact, in tracking my sleep, I've seen a straightforward correlation between when my last meal is and when I go to sleep. Eating late impacts my sleep quality and respective readiness and nervous system recovery the following day. Of course, there are times when I don't stick to this rule, but **those are the exceptions**, not the norm.

Generally, you want to eat your last lighter meal at least three hours prior to when you intend to go to sleep. Sadly this isn't what the majority of people do. Late night meals, snacking, and food consumption all contribute to poor impacts in high sleep quality.

11. ACCESSORIES AND SLEEP SUPPLEMENTS

A. Ear Plugs

An essential for me was getting used to sleeping with earplugs every night, regardless of my environment. You can adjust to continuous ambient sounds without plugs, but whenever there's a spike or unusual, irregular sound that impacts the sleep environment, earplugs do wonders to prevent that startle and dampen that. You will still hear your alarm because it is a proximity startle, but earplugs will do wonders to mitigate sounds that otherwise might wake you.

Earplugs come in many different forms, and I think the best choice is as simple as your preference. I actually opt for cheap disposable **Bright Honeywells** when sleeping. After a few weeks of use, they will lose their resiliency and become harder to fit in, but they work great and seem to stay in my ear canals well. NPR (noise protection rating) above 25 are usually quite sufficient, unless you're sleeping in a loud environment. Then I'd opt for something 32 and higher.

For going out to loud events (something I used to do a lot more often in my 20s and early 30s) I actually had **TRU Customs Westone earplugs** made several years ago that I still use. All in for around $300 you can get an audiologist to mold your ears and order a pair.

The advantage of these is they attenuate rather than simply dull the sounds. Attenuation lowers the overall sound decibel level without changing the sound stage. Whereas the Honeywell disposable plugs will dull out and alter sound frequencies, the TRU Customs will more accurately preserve the sound. You will see musicians wear these when performing to protect their hearing while still allowing them to hear their own pitch and range accurately. I find them very helpful for loud bars, clubs and music shows for protecting my long term hearing while still allowing me to hear and interact with my social companions.

(i) They come with inserts to adjust their NPR, which you can change in and out.
(ii) They can be made in skin colors that make them very low profile, barely noticeable.
(iii) They allow you to get a true sample of the sound in music shows and when conversing.

The only real downside is these earplugs are expensive at $100 / pop. One time I pulled one out while on a street corner, and it fell out of my hand and I lost it. I was able to replace it but that little mishap cost me a trip to the audiologist and $100.

B. Cooler Bed

I first heard about ChiliPads reading Tools of Titans by Tim Ferris. In his summary of overall things that top performers recommended, ChiliPad was near the top. It makes a difference. Would I say it's a game-changer? Probably. Can you sleep well without one, probably. I started sleeping with one in August 2019, and I've noticed my sleep is deeper. It is a large investment (+ $1,000) but I think it's worth it for most of us to seriously consider as it will add a level of comfort and coziness you would otherwise not experience.

If you're interested in learning more and getting discounts, you can check out my youtube videos from my channel where you'll see my in depth assessment of the product and how it works.

C. Eye Masks

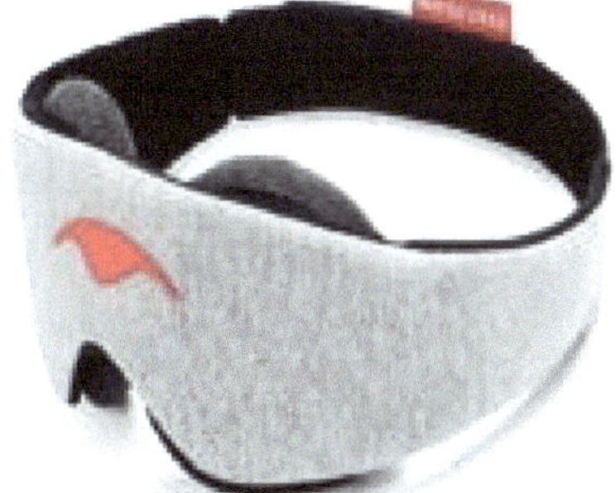

Image: Manta Sleep Mask

As mentioned above, I always sleep with an eye mask now. I do this primarily so I can avoid the stress and worry of having to blackout a room when I am not sleeping in my regular darkened sleep environment. By being used to sleeping with a mask, I find it reduces anxiety and concerns about light I might get in other rooms. Personally, I've found the Manta Eye Mask to be one of the best on the market. You don't have to use that, but I would recommend investing in one that:

(i) stays on your head,
(ii) is comfortable and
(iii) yields optimal light blocking.

The Manta Sleep Mask for me, does all three of these exceptionally well and is adjustable to fit different face shapes and sizes.

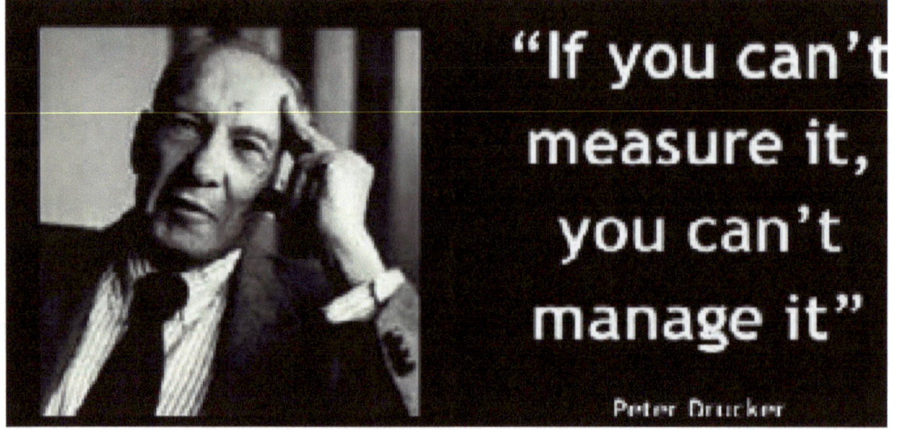

Trackers

"If you can't measure it, you can't manage it" - Peter Drucker. It seems so simple, but so many of us still do NOT track and manage arguably the single most important health variable, our sleep. Technology has evolved over the last decade, which has made it very easy and quite cost-effective to measure our sleep. When we measure something, it forces us to become more conscious of it, less ignorant to it, and improve.

OuraRing is my preferred biomarker for sleep tracking. It's low profile, and I find it to be quite accurate when comparing it with other trackers for observing my deep and REM sleep, as well as calculating my sleep efficiency and quality. That said, it's $300 and I realize for some that's a substantial amount to shell out for a biotracker you'll be using mainly for sleep tracking.

AutoSleep for Apple Watch is a popular one for those who already have, and are comfortable wearing, their Apple Watch while sleeping. Personally, the watch to me is a bit much for me to wear, but this is a $2.99 app that provides tracking insights you can get and start right away.

Whoop Band is another overall bio tracker that I've been testing out the past 60 days. It is lower profile than the watch but bigger than the ring. Whoop has some cool advantages to create more community. You can create groups with friends and teams to create accountability. It also seems to have a very well built dashboard to track athletic performance as well as recovery. I haven't looked fully into it, my experience is the OuraRing does a better job tracking my deep and REM sleep stages, but I'm still testing this out .It's an option for some with a $30/month option for bio / sleep tracking with the group option.

Here's a comparison between Oura vs Whoop's dashboard to show more specifics. I've also created a detailed review video comparing the two.

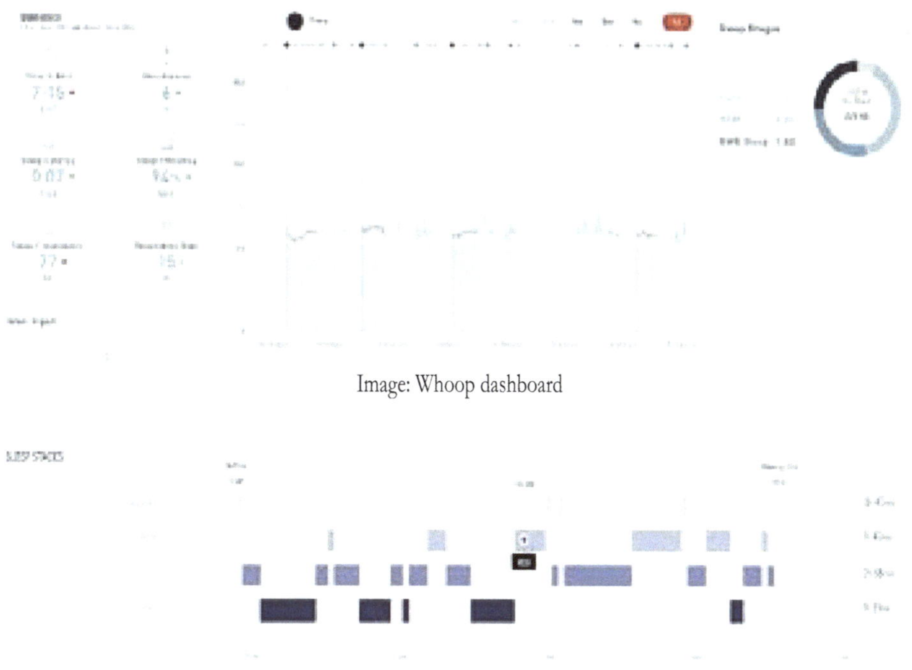

Image: Whoop dashboard

Image: Oura dashboard

One final note with trackers. Although ignorance is not bliss, perception of reality can play a powerful role in human psychology and our behavior. Tracking sleep can have a placebo effect on your overall daily performance. If you track a rough night of sleep, the tracker might reinforce for you to buy into a poor night of sleep being a sentence to write off that day.

To circumvent this impact on myself, I no longer review my sleep data upon waking. In my experience I've found it much more helpful to journal how I'm feeling in the morning, and then reflect on the actual data at the end of my day. Then I can think about the prior day, patterns, things I'm doing that are impacting the sleep I got that previous evening. Tracking is a very good thing, but you need to use the data, not let it use you.

Supplements

I'm not a big fan of supplements. I try and look at anything I take that alters my inner physiology as a crutch to reach a goal of not needing them, yet regularly using them. I am a fan of seeking out, and doing the things naturally that are more ancestrally consistent with what our body needs to thrive without supplementing "crutches."

If I use a supplement, I always look for ways to do so to fuel the source of micronutrients that feed my body's sleep process. Rather than take a hormone, I prefer to take the building blocks my body needs to produce that hormone.

That said, below are a few hacks I've found over the years. I know we're all coming from different places of being able to fall asleep quickly, as well as sleeping throughout our nights. Supplements can be a great tool to help get us to where we want to finally be, but they should not be the final answer.

Melatonin

Many individuals like to take exogenous melatonin. I'm not a big fan of using this long term and prefer supplementing precursors to hormones because some research shows that supplementing an actual hormone can interrupt the body's long term ability to produce that hormone.

Fortunately, many studies have been conducted, and the overall consensus is fairly strong that taking melatonin even weekly hasn't shown adverse effects on natural hormone production.

If I'm up very late, multiple hours past my regular sleep time, or if I'm traveling across time zones, I will usually take melatonin. With travel, or sleep whenever I'm more than a few hours outside my normal window of sleeping, I'll utilize melatonin or some other sleep aid (I'll mention more below) to help boost the hormone signaling in my body to produce adequate sleep pressure.

With melatonin the dosing is more optimal at 0.3mg vs. the typically 3-5mg you see in over the counter supplements.

With melatonin the dosing is more optimal at 0.3mg vs. the typically 3-5mg you see in over the counter supplements. I use Sundown brand because it's well-rated and gives me the dosing I want. Melatonin is cheap, but I would be wary of needing to take it all the time and look for addressing - as we have covered many sections in this book - the root cause of why you need it to sleep.

New Mood

I've been a fan of ONNIT nutrition supplements lately. I've dabbled with a few other sleep supplements to see if I can bump up my efficiency, but in my experience, most leave me either not sleeping much better or waking up super groggy. The New Mood works well for me and seems to hit the sweet spot.

I prefer the quality and ingredients used in the New Mood supplement.I've tested several of their other products and am now affiliated with ONNIT. Use code "karnivore" at checkout for 10% off and give their products a try. New Mood is one that I've dabbled with at different doses and noticed some direct impacts on my ability to sleep more easily and deeper.

If I'm having a particular off schedule sleep and, or, I am wound up, I will usually go to New Mood. If I am traveling and farther than a few hours off my usual schedule, I'll usually go to melatonin. And in those rare cases where I'm up till near sunrise I'll combine them both.

12. The Action Plan

Alright, we've covered a lot. I've given you essentially all that is known about how to optimize and sleep better. At this point I want to shift gears and in this section I'm going to coach you through a progression of how I treat my own case of insomnia. What to do, when to do it and how you might start to improve your sleep.

Now this section could become an entire book itself. There's just so many unique cases and places people are coming from to treat their sleep challenges. But for our purposes I'm going to guide you through the best, most impactful and easiest ways to build momentum to improve this aspect of your sleep. Plan to make these changes over several weeks, perhaps adding something each week. Human behavior and habits have momentum, changing all at once usually results in failure of all, but slowly adjusting some will result in long term consistency.

If you downloaded our free progress guide you'll have a solid workflow you can get started on. But since you've purchased this book I want to give you a lot of the keys here so you have it all in one place.

I've listed these in order, based on the average individual and ease of implementation, that I think most would benefit from.

I. Mental Game

I've talked about how important it is to master this component, how little others address it. The power of the human mind, cannot be under-stated. If you can program new beliefs to believe you will sleep better, not become anxious when going to sleep, it will do wonders to tremendously improve your overall sleep.

This is the single most important thing you should focus on if you have any doubts that you will not sleep exceptionally well when going to bed.

a. Reread the section above and ensure that you have a foundational understanding
b. Write down at least 2, if not 3 affirmations per night. Do this starting tonight
c. Keep this a consistent practice (it will take 2-3 mins).
d. Stay consistent with affirmations for 21 days at which point you can decide to change.

II. Adjust the days activities

a. Are you getting movement?
b. Are you getting outside, getting sunlight earlier in the day to start your clock?
c. Are you eating a meal earlier in your day?

All these things will kick start your body's natural clock and circadian rhythm to know the day has begun and will help your body later on to know it's completed the cycle and it's time to power down.

III. Cycling down obstacles

a. Several hours prior to bed, are you reducing blue light shifting to more red?
b. Are you minimizing screen brightness and exposure after sunset?
c. Are you lowering the temperature in your home?
d. Are you lowering the intensity of stress and intense thinking?
e. Add stretching and light audiobooks into your evening routine. They release physical and emotional stress to support easier transition into sleep.

Our ancestors had fire and moonlight. Both of these were much lower and much more limited in intensity than the last 150 years of blue light we've experienced. When the human body isn't physically experiencing signals it's evolved to experience, it can be more challenging to sleep. Change out the master bath bulb for a red low wattage one. Get adjustable lights to change brightness and use programs like f.lux to turn screen light warmer.

IV. Consumption Limitations

a. Cut back on uppers and coffee as the sun goes down.
b. Remember coffee can stay in your system for days, consider limiting or totally eliminating it. (I know this is a big one - so if you don't want to that's fine) but it will affect your ability to sleep deeper and fall asleep quicker. There's also a lot of problems with coffee beyond the scope of this book.
c. Alcohol, marijuana. Again these molecules may seem to help us sleep but they can be quite damaging to our body's ability to actually sleep well. Consider cutting back.
d. Push your evening meals earlier on days when it's socially acceptable and convenient.

13. CONCLUSION

Sleep is such an undervalued part of our health and modern society. It is one of the biggest levers to optimal human performance, both physically and mentally. It is our natural way to recover and heal. It is when we process our thinking and flush toxins from our brains. It is a place where our mind synthesizes and activates creative problem-solving.

With the invention of electricity only 150 years ago, modern society has significantly changed the way humans were evolved to sleep. Most of us are confusing our biology with artificially stable room temperatures, light spectrums, and nnEMF waves we've never ancestrally experienced after sundown.

150 years isn't even a blip on the 20M year evolutionary timeline we evolved from. Yet in that blink, we've drastically changed how we live, consuming media, food, and light in ways entirely unnatural for our biology. It's no surprise the levels of mental and physical disease we've seen have exploded.

We drastically limited and deprioritized our body's signaling and ability to recover, process, and restore us. After years of these patterns, we develop behaviors and limiting beliefs and accept the new diminished level of health, function, and ability to sleep easily.

The good news is we can get back to our roots quite quickly. We can learn to respect our hominid ancestors by creating and developing new simple habits. Though habit change is not easy, most of what allows us to take control of our core health is really about letting go, reprogramming bad beliefs, and making simple changes.

I firmly believe that if you follow the steps outlined in this book, your health will drastically improve. I believe it will change for the better, and you will start noticing how much more productive and vital you feel. You will reverse disease, mood, mental illness, and have much more strength and energy. It is one of, if not the biggest component to optimal human health. Along with diet, light, and movement, respecting these pillars of who we are as humans, we can take control of our health and vitality.

Thank you for investing in your health. I'm grateful I could serve as a guide on this journey. I look forward to hearing how your journey unfolds, please share it with me and the world and encourage others to prioritize it as a key pillar to leading a vital and healthy life.

Let's get optimized!

14. REFERENCES

01 Oura. (2019, April). Knowing the Stages of Sleep Will Help You Know Yourself. Here's Why. https://landing.ouraring.com/ln1d-stages-of-sleep

02 Rettner, R. (2013, May 20). Live Science. Sleep-Deprived Teen Drivers More Likely to Crash. https://www.livescience.com/34520-young-drivers-sleep-car-crashes.html

03 Ellenbogen, J.M. (2005, April 12). Cognitive benefits of sleep and their loss due to sleep deprivation. https://www.ncbi.nlm.nih.gov/pubmed/15824327

04 Landrigan, C.P., Rothschild, J.M., Cronin, J.W., Kaushal, R., Burdick, E., Katz, J.T., Lilly, C.M., Stone, P.H., Lockley, S.W., Bates, D.W. & Czeisler, C.A. (2004, October 28). Effect of reducing interns' work hours on serious medical errors in intensive care units. https://www.ncbi.nlm.nih.gov/pubmed/15509817

05 Williamson, A.M. & Feyer, A.M. (2000, October). Moderate sleep deprivation produces impairments in cognitive and motor performance equivalent to legally prescribed levels of alcohol intoxication. https://www.ncbi.nlm.nih.gov/pubmed/10984335

06 Walker, M.P., Liston, C., Hobson, J.A. & Stickgold, R. (2002, November 14). Cognitive flexibility across the sleep-wake cycle: REM-sleep enhancement of anagram problem solving. https://www.ncbi.nlm.nih.gov/pubmed/12421655

07 Könen, T., Dirk, J. & Schmiedek, F. (2015, February). Cognitive benefits of last night's sleep: daily variations in children's sleep behavior are related to working memory fluctuations. https://www.ncbi.nlm.nih.gov/pubmed/25052368

08 Mednick, S.C., Makovski, T., Cai, D.J. & Jiang, Y.V. (2009, October). leep and rest facilitate implicit memory in a visual search task. https://www.ncbi.nlm.nih.gov/pubmed/19379769

09 Tsuno, N., Besset, A. & Ritchie, K. (2005, October). Sleep and depression. https://www.ncbi.nlm.nih.gov/pubmed/16259539

10 Bernert, R.A., Turvey, C.L., Conwell, Y. & Joiner, T.E Jr. (2014, October 7). Association of poor subjective sleep quality with risk for death by suicide during a 10-year period: a longitudinal, population-based study of late life. https://www.ncbi.nlm.nih.gov/pubmed/25133759

11 Hayley, A.C., Williams, L.J., Venugopal, K., Kennedy, G.A., Berk, M. & Pasco, J.A. (2015, February). The relationships between insomnia, sleep apnoea and depression: findings from the American National Health and Nutrition Examination Survey, 2005-2008. https://www.ncbi.nlm.nih.gov/pubmed/25128225

12 Cappuccio, F.P., Cooper, D., D'Elia, L., Strazzullo, P. & Miller, M.A. (2011, June). leep duration predicts cardiovascular outcomes: a systematic review and meta-analsis of prospective studies. https://www.ncbi.nlm.nih.gov/pubmed/21300732

13 Mah, C.D., Mah, K.E., Kezirian, E.J. & Dement, W.C. (2011, July 1). he effects of sleep extension on the athletic performance of collegiate basketball players. https://www.ncbi.nlm.nih.gov/pubmed/21731144

14 Goldman, S.E., Stone, K.L, Ancoli-Israel, S., Blackwell, T., Ewing, S.K., Boudreau, R., Cauley, J.A., Hall, M., Matthews, K.A. & Newman, A.B. (2007, October 30). Poor sleep is associated with poorer physical performance and greater functional limitations in older women. https://www.ncbi.nlm.nih.gov/pubmed/17969465

15 Kirchheimer, S. (2003, October 1). How Sleep Affects Cancer. Poor Sleep Alters Hormones That Influence Cancer Cells. https://www.webmd.com/cancer/news/20031001/how-sleep-affects-cancer#1

16 American Psychological Association. (n.d.). Stress and Sleep. https://www.apa.org/news/press/releases/stress/2013/sleep

17 Tauseef, A., James, C., Ahmed, A., Theodore, L.W. & William, C.O. (2013, December 28). Sleep, immunity and inflammation in gastrointestinal disorders. https://www.ncbi.nlm.nih.gov/pmc/articles/PMC3882397/

18 Jami, A.K. MD, David, T.R. MD & Tauseef, A. MD. (2013, November 9). Sleep and Inflammatory Bowel Disease: Exploring the Relationship Between Sleep Disturbances and Inflammation. https://www.ncbi.nlm.nih.gov/pmc/articles/PMC3995194/

19 American Academy of Sleep Medicine. (2008, June 9). Sleep Extension Improves Alertness And Performance During And Following Subsequent Sleep Restriction.https://w ww.sciencedaily.com/releases/2008/06/080609071213.htm

20 Sanjay, R.P. & Frank, B.H. (2012 , September 6). Short Sleep Duration and Weight Gain: A Systematic Review. https://onlinelibrary.wiley.com/doi/full/10.1038/oby.2007.118

21 Shahrad, T., Ling, L., Diane, A., Terry, Y. & Emmanuel, M. (2004, December 7). Short Sleep Duration Is Associated with Reduced Leptin, Elevated Ghrelin, and Increased Body Mass Index. https://www.ncbi.nlm.nih.gov/pmc/articles/PMC535701/

22 SleepFoundation.org. (n.d.). Sleep, Athletic Performance, and Recovery. https://www.sleepfoundation.org/articles/sleep-athletic-performance-and-recovery

23 Louise, H. (2016, March 22). Mirror Work: 21 Days to Heal Your Life. https://www.amazon.com/Mirror-Work-Days-Heal-Your/dp/1401949827

24 Wikipedia. (2019, January 22). Hay House. https://en.wikipedia.org/wiki/Hay_House

25 Arlene, S. MS, RD. (2017, February 10). The Top 10 Benefits of Regular Exercise. https://www.healthline.com/nutrition/10-benefits-of-exercise#section10

26 Mercola. (2020, January 19). Why You Should Embrace Healthful Sun Exposure. https://articles.mercola.com/sites/articles/archive/2020/01/19/sun-exposure-health-benefits.aspx

27 Mancebo, S.E. & Wang, S.Q. (2014). Skin cancer: role of ultraviolet radiation in carcinogenesis. https://www.ncbi.nlm.nih.gov/pubmed/25252745

28 Ristic, A. MS. (2020, January 6). 10 Benefits of Cold Exposure & Cold Showers + Precautions. https://selfhacked.com/blog/12-reasons-embrace-cold/

29 Marbach, T. (2019, June 6). HOW TO SUPERCHARGE YOUR DEEP SLEEP. https://www.wimhofmethod.com/blog/how-to-supercharge-your-deep-sleep

30 Azqueta, A. & Collins, A. (2016, December 8). Polyphenols and DNA Damage: A Mixed Blessing. https://www.ncbi.nlm.nih.gov/pmc/articles/PMC5188440/

31 Gunnars, K. BSc. (2019, January 28). Mycotoxins Myth: The Truth About Mold in Coffee. https://www.healthline.com/nutrition/the-mycotoxins-in-coffee-myth#safe-production-methods

32 Science Daily. (2016, October 17). Does weed help you sleep? Probably not. https://www.sciencedaily.com/releases/2016/10/161017155004.htm

33 Yetish, G., Kaplan, H., Gurven, M., Wood, B., Pontzer, H., Manger, P.R., Wilson, C., McGregor, R. & Siegel, J.M. (2015, October 15). Natural Sleep and Its Seasonal Variations in Three Pre-industrial Societies. https://www.cell.com/current-biology/fulltext/S0960-9822(15)01157-4

34 Cho, C., Yoon, H., Kang, S., Kim, L., Lee, E. & Lee, H. (2018, May 15). Impact of Exposure to Dim Light at Night on Sleep in Female and Comparison with Male Subjects. https://www.ncbi.nlm.nih.gov/pmc/articles/PMC5976009/

35 Robin, A. (2019, June 10). Sleeping with artificial light at night associated with weight gain in women. https://www.nih.gov/news-events/news-releases/sleeping-artificial-light-night-associated-weight-gain-women

36 Wikipidea. (2020, March 25). Control of fire by early humans. https://simple.wikipedia.org/wiki/Control_of_fire_by_early_humans

37 Gillihan, S.J. Ph.D. (2019, October 14). Want to Sleep Better? Go for a Walk. https://www.psychologytoday.com/us/blog/think-act-be/201910/want-sleep-better-go-walk

38 Kogevinas, M., Espinosa, A., Castelló, A., Gómez, I.., Guevara, M., Martin, V., Amiano, P., Alguacil, J., Peiro, R., Moreno, V., Costas, L., Fernández, G., Jimenez, J.J., Marcos, R.,Gomez, B., Llorca, J., Moreno, C., Fernández, T., Oribe, M., Aragones, N., Papantoniou, K., Pollán, M., Castano, G. and Romaguera, D. (2018, July 17). Effect of mistimed eating patterns on breast and prostate cancer risk (MCC-Spain Study). https://onlinelibrary.wiley.com/doi/full/10.1002/ijc.31649

39 Baron, K.G. PhD. MPH., Reid, K.J. PhD., Van Horn, L. PhD, RD. & Zee, P.C. MD, PhD. (2012, October 2). Contribution of evening macronutrient intake to total caloric intake and body mass index. https://www.ncbi.nlm.nih.gov/pmc/articles/PMC3640498/

40 Baron, K.G. PhD. MPH., Reid, K.J. PhD., Kern, A.S. & Zee, P.C. MD, PhD. (2012, September 10). Contribution of evening macronutrient intake to total caloric intake and body mass index. https://onlinelibrary.wiley.com/doi/full/10.1038/oby.2011.100

www.ingramcontent.com/pod-product-compliance
Lightning Source LLC
Chambersburg PA
CBHW040131270326
41928CB00004B/67